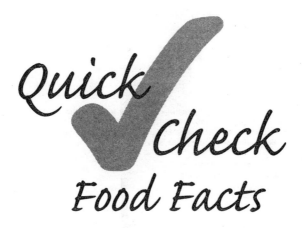

Quick ✓ Check
Food Facts

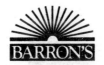

BARRON'S

All inquiries should be addressed to:
Barron's Educational Series, Inc.
250 Wireless Boulevard
Hauppauge, New York 11788
http://www.barronseduc.com

International Standard Book No. 0-7641-0874-3

Library of Congress Catalog Card No. 98-25679

Library of Congress Cataloging-in-Publication Data
Quick Check Food Facts / editorial staff of Barron's Educational
  Series, Inc.
    p.   cm.
  ISBN 0-7641-0874-3 (Large edition) ISBN 0-7641-0754-2 (Mini edition)
  1. Food—Composition—Tables.   2. Nutrition—Tables. I. Barron's
Educational Series, Inc.
TX551.B525   1998
613.2'8—dc21   98-25679
                                                                  CIP

PRINTED IN THE UNITED STATES OF AMERICA
9 8 7 6 5 4

Contents

Preface

The information in this book is based on the *USDA Nutrient Database for Standard Reference, Release 11-1*, published in computer-readable form by the U.S. Department of Agriculture. The original database is very large and unwieldy, and we have extracted just the most useful information for publication here.

For each food, we list serving size, and then, per serving:

Total calories	Fat (grams;)
Calories from fat	Cholesterol (milligrams)
Protein (grams)	Sodium (milligrams)
Carbohydrates (grams)	Fiber (grams)

Calories from fat were computed from factors given in the USDA database. The number of calories per gram of fat is approximately 9 but varies somewhat depending on the type of food. In a very few cases, numbers were missing from the USDA database. They are left blank here.

Introduction

Can You Judge Food by Its Label?

In response to the public's demand for more information, the Food and Drug Administration (FDA) has set mandatory nutrition labeling requirements for food manufacturers. Nearly all processed foods must display a label of "Nutrition Facts." This information has been designed to take the guesswork out of grocery shopping, to help consumers choose more healthful foods, and to offer an incentive to food manufacturers to improve the nutritional quality of their products.

Look to the Label

Listed under "Nutrition Facts" is the information you need to compare foods and make informed choices. Food labels indicate serving size; calorie content; the amounts of carbohydrate, protein, fat, cholesterol, and sodium; and the content of four important nutrients — vitamin A, vitamin C, iron, and calcium. Also, you can review the label to determine the exact ingredients — keeping in mind that the largest ingredient by weight is listed first.

While food labels can make it easier to keep track of what you are eating, they can also help you stay within the U.S. Dietary Guidelines. These guidelines recommend that 55–60% of daily calories should come from carbohydrates, 30% or less from fat, and 10–15% from protein.

Can Serving Size Make a Difference?

When reading labels, pay close attention to serving size. Serving sizes that now appear on food labels are more realistic than in the past and tend to represent how much an average person eats. Serving sizes are broken down into household measures such as cups, tablespoons, ounces or amounts such as one cookie or one slice of bread.

Nevertheless, serving size is one of the more difficult concepts to keep in mind. For example, a serving size of potato chips is about a handful. However, does anyone really eat just one handful?

How Can You Use Percent Daily Value to Help Build a Healthful Diet?

Once you are familiar with serving sizes, the next bit of important information to look at is the reference numbers on the nutrition label. The amount of nutrients, in grams or milligrams of fat, carbohydrates, protein, cholesterol, and sodium, must be listed. However, Percent Daily Values are also indicated. These reference numbers give a general idea of a food's nutrient contribution to the total daily diet. Daily Values are listed for people who eat 2,000 calories a day. This level was chosen, in part, because it approximates the caloric requirements of postmenopausal women who tend to have the highest excessive intake of calories and fat. Daily Values for people who eat 2,500 calories per day may also be listed.

You can use Percent Daily Values to compare foods and to see if your diet fits within the current dietary recommendations. If you typically eat 2,000 calories a day, you can total up the Percent Daily Values of dietary fat that you eat in a day. If it adds up to 100%, then your diet fits with the recommendations for fat.

Nutrition Tip: For fat, saturated fat, and cholesterol, choose foods that have a low Percent Daily Value. For total carbohydrate, dietary fiber, vitamins, and iron, you should try to achieve 100% of the Daily Value each day. For these nutrients, try to select foods that have a high Percent Daily Value.

What Are Nutrient Content Claims?

A nutrient content claim is a word or phrase on a food label that helps describe the amount of nutrients in a food. These key words and nutrient claims are defined by the government. For instance:

- **Free:** The product contains none or a very small amount of a component. Calorie-free is fewer than 5 calories per serving; fat-free is less than 0.5 gram per serving.

- **Low:** Low can be used on foods that can be eaten frequently without exceeding dietary guidelines for one or more of these components: fat, cholesterol, sodium, and calories. Low-fat is 3 grams or less per serving; low-sodium is 140 milligrams or less per serving; low-cholesterol is 20 milligrams or less per serving and 2 grams or less saturated fat per serving; low-calorie is less than 40 calories per serving.

- **High:** This can be used if the food contains 20% or more of the Daily Value for a particular nutrient.

- **Good Source:** This can be used on foods containing 10–19% of the Daily Value of a particular nutrient.

- **Light (Lite):** This can be used on foods containing one-third less calories or no more than one-half the fat of the higher calorie, high-fat version; or no more than one-half the sodium of the higher sodium version.

Consumers have been flooded with information regarding the relationship between diet and the prevention of disease. Reading food labels and using references such as *Quick Check Food Facts* can help you make informed choices and help reduce the risk of disease. Once you become label literate, nutrient values and daily percentages will not seem so overwhelming. Keep in mind that the best approach to healthful eating is to eat foods at each meal that contain a small portion of everything rather than saving up your fat grams for a big splurge at dessert!

Carolyn E. Moore

Vegetables and Vegetable Products

Food Serving size	Cal.	Fat cal.	Prot.	Carb.	Fat	Chol.	Sod.	Fiber
Alfalfa seeds, sprouted, raw 1 tablespoon (3g)	1	0	0	0	0	0	0	0.1
Artichokes, (globe or french), boiled, drained, without salt $\frac{1}{2}$ cup hearts (84g)	42	0	3	9	0	0	80	4.2
Artichokes, (globe or french), frozen, boiled, drained, without salt 1 cup (168g)	76	0	5	15	0	0	89	8.4
Arugula, raw 1 leaf (2g)	1	0	0	0	0	0	1	0.0
Asparagus, boiled, drained 4 spears, ($\frac{1}{2}''$ base) (60g)	14	0	2	2	0	0	7	1.2
Asparagus, canned, drained solids 1 spear (about 5" long) (18g)	3	2	0	0	0	0	52	0.4
Asparagus, frozen, boiled, drained, without salt 1 cup (180g)	50	0	5	9	0	0	7	3.6
Bamboo shoots, boiled, drained, without salt 1 cup, ($\frac{1}{2}''$ slices) (120g)	14	0	2	2	0	0	5	1.2
Bamboo shoots, canned, drained solids 1 cup ($\frac{1}{8}''$ slices) (131g)	25	0	3	4	0	0	9	1.3

1

Food Serving size	Cal.	Fat cal.	Prot.	Carb.	Fat	Chol.	Sod.	Fiber
Beet greens, boiled, drained, without salt $\frac{1}{2}$ cup, 1″ pieces (72g)	19	0	2	4	0	0	174	2.2
Beets, boiled, drained $\frac{1}{2}$ cup slices (85g)	37	0	2	9	0	0	65	1.7
Beets, canned, drained solids 1 cup, diced (157g)	49	0	2	11	0	0	305	3.1
Beets, Harvard, canned, solids and liquids 1 cup, slices (246g)	180	0	2	44	0	0	399	4.9
Beets, pickled, canned, solids and liquids 1 cup, slices (227g)	148	0	2	36	0	0	599	
Borage, boiled, drained, without salt 100 grams	25	8	2	4	1	0	88	
Broadbeans, immature seeds, boiled, drained, without salt 100 grams	62	0	5	10	0	0	41	4.0
Broccoli, boiled, drained, without salt 1 medium stalk ($7\frac{1}{2}″- 8″$ long) (180g)	50	0	5	9	0	0	47	5.4
Broccoli, Chinese, cooked 1 cup (88g)	19	7	1	4	1	0	6	1.8
Broccoli, frozen, chopped, boiled, drained, without salt 1 cup (184g)	52	0	6	9	0	0	44	5.5
Broccoli, frozen, spears, boiled, drained, without salt $\frac{1}{2}$ cup (92g)	26	0	3	5	0	0	22	2.8
Broccoli, raw 1 cup, flowerets (71g)	20	0	2	4	0	0	19	2.1
Brussels sprouts, boiled, drained, without salt 1 sprout (21g)	8	2	1	2	0	0	4	0.6
Brussels sprouts, frozen, boiled, drained, without salt 1 cup (155g)	65	0	6	12	0	0	36	6.2
Cabbage, boiled, drained, without salt $\frac{1}{2}$ cup shredded (75g)	17	0	1	3	0	0	6	1.5
Cabbage, Chinese (pak-choi), boiled, drained, without salt 1 cup, shredded (170g)	20	0	3	3	0	0	58	3.4

Food Serving size	Cal.	Fat cal.	Prot.	Carb.	Fat	Chol.	Sod.	Fiber
Cabbage, Chinese (pak-choi), raw								
1 cup, shredded (70g)	9	0	1	1	0	0	46	0.7
Cabbage, Chinese (pe-tsai), boiled, drained, without salt								
1 leaf (14g)	2	0	0	0	0	0	1	0.4
Cabbage, Chinese (pe-tsai), raw								
1 cup, shredded (76g)	12	0	1	2	0	0	7	2.3
Cabbage, raw								
1 cup, shredded (70g)	18	0	1	4	0	0	13	1.4
Cabbage, red, boiled, drained, without salt								
1 leaf (22g)	5	0	0	1	0	0	2	0.4
Cabbage, red, raw								
1 cup, shredded (70g)	19	0	1	4	0	0	8	1.4
Cabbage, Savoy, boiled, drained, without salt								
1 cup, shredded (145g)	35	0	3	7	0	0	35	4.3
Cabbage, Savoy, raw								
1 cup, shredded (70g)	19	0	1	4	0	0	20	2.1
Carrot juice, canned								
1 fl oz (30g)	12	0	0	3	0	0	9	0.3
Carrots, baby, raw								
1 medium (10g)	4	1	0	1	0	0	4	0.2
Carrots, boiled, drained, without salt								
1 tablespoon (10g)	5	0	0	1	0	0	7	0.3
Carrots, canned, regular pack, drained solids								
1 cup, sliced (146g)	37	0	1	9	0	0	353	2.9
Carrots, frozen, boiled, drained, without salt								
1 cup, sliced (146g)	53	0	1	12	0	0	86	5.8
Carrots, raw								
1 cup, grated (110g)	47	0	1	11	0	0	39	3.3
Catsup								
1 tablespoon (15g)	16	0	0	4	0	0	178	0.2
Cauliflower, boiled, drained, without salt								
3 flowerets (54g)	12	0	1	2	0	0	8	1.6

Food Serving size	Cal.	Fat cal.	Prot.	Carb.	Fat	Chol.	Sod.	Fiber
Cauliflower, frozen, boiled, drained, without salt 1 cup, (1″ pieces) (180g)	34	0	4	7	0	0	32	5.4
Cauliflower, raw 1 floweret (13g)	3	0	0	1	0	0	4	0.3
Celery, boiled, drained, without salt 2 stalks (75g)	14	0	1	3	0	0	68	1.5
Celery, raw 1 cup, diced (120g)	19	0	1	5	0	0	104	2.4
Chard, Swiss, boiled, drained, without salt 1 cup, chopped (175g)	35	0	4	7	0	0	313	3.5
Chard, Swiss, raw 1 cup (36g)	7	0	1	1	0	0	77	0.7
Chives, raw 1 teaspoon, chopped (1g)	0	0	0	0	0	0	0	0.0
Cilantro, raw 1 teaspoon (2g)	0	0	0	0	0	0	1	0.1
Coleslaw 1 tablespoon (8g)	6	0	0	1	0	1	2	0.2
Collards, boiled, drained, without salt 1 cup, chopped (190g)	49	0	4	10	0	0	17	5.7
Corn, sweet, yellow, boiled, drained, without salt 1 baby ear (8g)	9	1	0	2	0	0	1	0.2
Corn, sweet, yellow, canned, cream style, regular pack 1 cup (256g)	184	0	5	46	0	0	730	2.6
Corn, sweet, yellow, canned, whole kernel, drained solids 1 cup (164g)	133	14	5	31	2	0	351	3.3
Corn, sweet, yellow, frozen, kernels cut off cob, boiled, drained, without salt $\frac{1}{2}$ cup (82g)	66	0	2	16	0	0	4	1.6
Corn with red and green peppers, canned, solids and liquids 1 cup (227g)	170	19	5	41	2	0	788	
Cress, garden, boiled, drained, without salt $\frac{1}{2}$ cup (68g)	16	6	1	3	1	0	5	0.7

Food Serving size	Cal.	Fat cal.	Prot.	Carb.	Fat	Chol.	Sod.	Fiber
Cress, garden, raw 1 sprig (1g)	0	0	0	0	0	0	0	0.0
Cucumber, peeled, raw 1 cup, sliced (119g)	14	0	1	2	0	0	2	1.2
Cucumber, with peel, raw $\frac{1}{2}$ cup slices (52g)	7	0	1	2	0	0	1	0.5
Dandelion greens, boiled, drained, without salt 1 cup, chopped (105g)	35	9	2	6	1	0	46	3.2
Dandelion greens, raw 1 cup, chopped (55g)	25	5	2	5	1	0	42	2.2
Eggplant, boiled, drained, without salt 1 cup, (1" cubes) (99g)	28	0	1	7	0	0	3	2.0
Eggplant, raw 1 cup, cubes (82g)	21	0	1	5	0	0	2	1.6
Endive, raw $\frac{1}{2}$ cup, chopped (25g)	4	0	0	1	0	0	6	0.8
Fennel, bulb, raw 1 cup, sliced (87g)	27	0	1	6	0	0	45	2.6
Garlic, raw 1 teaspoon (3g)	4	0	0	1	0	0	1	0.1
Ginger root, raw 1 teaspoon (2g)	1	0	0	0	0	0	0	0.0
Grape leaves, canned 1 leaf (4g)	3	1	0	0	0	0	114	
Grape leaves, raw 1 leaf (3g)	3	1	0	1	0	0	0	0.3
Hearts of palm, canned 1 piece (33g)	9	3	1	2	0	0	141	0.7
Hyacinth-beans, immature seeds, boiled, drained, without salt 1 cup (87g)	44	0	3	8	0	0	2	
Jerusalem artichokes, raw 1 cup, slices (150g)	114	0	3	26	0	0	6	3.0
Kale, boiled, drained, without salt 1 cup, chopped (130g)	36	0	3	8	0	0	30	2.6

Food Serving size	Cal.	Fat cal.	Prot.	Carb.	Fat	Chol.	Sod.	Fiber
Kohlrabi, boiled, drained, without salt								
1 cup, sliced (165g)	48	0	3	12	0	0	35	1.6
Leeks (bulb and lower leaf-portion), boiled, drained, without salt								
$\frac{1}{4}$ cup chopped or								
diced (26g)	8	0	0	2	0	0	3	0.3
Leeks (bulb and lower leaf-portion), raw								
1 cup (89g)	54	0	2	12	0	0	18	1.8
Lemon grass (citronella), raw								
1 tablespoon (5g)	5	0	0	1	0	0	0	
Lentils, sprouted, stir-fried, without salt								
100 grams	101	0	9	21	0	0	10	
Lettuce, butterhead (includes Boston and bibb types), raw								
1 cup, shredded or								
chopped (55g)	7	0	1	1	0	0	3	0.6
Lettuce, cos or romaine, raw								
1 innerleaf (10g)	1	0	0	0	0	0	1	0.2
Lettuce, iceberg (includes crisphead types), raw								
1 cup, shredded or								
chopped (55g)	7	0	1	1	0	0	5	0.6
Lettuce, looseleaf, raw								
1 leaf (10g)	2	0	0	0	0	0	1	0.2
Lotus root, boiled, drained, without salt								
$\frac{1}{2}$ cup (60g)	40	0	1	10	0	0	27	1.8
Mountain yam, Hawaii, steamed, without salt								
1 cup, cubes (145g)	119	0	3	29	0	0	17	
Mountain yam, Hawaii, raw								
$\frac{1}{2}$ cup cubes (68g)	46	0	1	11	0	0	9	
Mushroom, oyster, raw								
1 small (15g)	6	1	1	1	0	0	5	0.3
Mushrooms, boiled, drained, without salt								
1 tablespoon (10g)	3	0	0	1	0	0	0	0.2
Mushrooms, canned, drained solids								
1 can (132g)	32	0	3	7	0	0	561	2.6
Mushrooms, enoki, raw								
1 medium (3g)	1	0	0	0	0	0	0	0.1

Food Serving size	Cal.	Fat cal.	Prot.	Carb.	Fat	Chol.	Sod.	Fiber
Mushrooms, raw 1 cup, pieces or slices (70g)	18	0	1	4	0	0	3	0.7
Mushrooms, shiitake, cooked, without salt 4 mushrooms (72g)	40	0	1	10	0	0	3	1.4
Mushrooms, shiitake, dried 1 mushroom (4g)	12	0	0	3	0	0	1	0.5
Mushrooms, straw, canned, drained solids 1 piece (6g)	2	1	0	0	0	0	23	0.1
Mustard greens, boiled, drained, without salt 1 cup, chopped (140g)	21	0	3	3	0	0	22	2.8
Mustard spinach, (tendergreen), boiled, drained, without salt 1 cup, chopped (180g)	29	0	4	5	0	0	25	3.6
New Zealand spinach, boiled, drained, without salt 1 cup, chopped (180g)	22	0	2	4	0	0	193	
New Zealand spinach, raw 1 cup, chopped (56g)	8	0	1	1	0	0	73	
Okra, boiled, drained, without salt ½ cup slices (80g)	26	0	2	6	0	0	4	1.6
Onion rings, breaded, par fried, frozen, prepared, heated in oven 1 cup (48g)	195	114	2	18	13	0	180	0.5
Onions, boiled, drained, without salt 1 tablespoon, chopped (15g)	7	0	0	2	0	0	0	0.2
Onions, canned, solids and liquids 1 onion (63g)	12	0	1	3	0	0	234	0.6
Onions, raw 1 cup, sliced (115g)	44	0	1	10	0	0	3	2.3
Parsley, raw 1 tablespoon (4g)	1	0	0	0	0	0	2	0.1
Parsnips, boiled, drained, without salt ½ cup slices (78g)	63	0	1	16	0	0	8	3.1
Peas and carrots, canned, regular pack, solids and liquids 1 cup (255g)	97	0	5	20	0	0	663	5.1

Food Serving size	Cal.	Fat cal.	Prot.	Carb.	Fat	Chol.	Sod.	Fiber
Peas and carrots, frozen, boiled, drained, without salt								
$\frac{1}{2}$ cup (80g)	38	0	2	8	0	0	54	2.4
Peas and onions, canned, solids and liquids								
1 cup (120g)	61	0	4	11	0	0	530	2.4
Peas and onions, frozen, boiled, drained, without salt								
1 cup (180g)	81	0	5	16	0	0	67	3.6
Peas, edible-podded, boiled, drained, without salt								
1 cup (160g)	67	0	5	11	0	0	6	4.8
Peas, green, boiled, drained, without salt								
1 cup (160g)	134	0	8	26	0	0	5	9.6
Peas, green, canned, regular pack, drained solids								
1 cup (170g)	117	0	7	22	0	0	428	6.8
Peas, mature seeds, sprouted, boiled, drained, without salt								
100 grams	118	8	7	22	1	0	3	
Pepper, ancho, dried								
1 pepper (17g)	48	11	2	9	1	0	7	3.7
Pepper, serrano, raw								
1 pepper (6g)	2	0	0	0	0	0	1	0.2
Peppers, chili, green, canned								
1 cup (139g)	29	0	1	7	0	0	552	2.8
Peppers, hot chili, green, canned, pods, excluding seeds, solids and liquids								
$\frac{1}{2}$ cup chopped or diced (68g)	14	0	1	3	0	0	798	0.7
Peppers, hot chili, green, raw								
1 pepper (45g)	18	0	1	4	0	0	3	0.9
Peppers, hot chile, sun-dried								
1 pepper (1g)	3	1	0	1	0	0	1	0.3
Peppers, jalapeno, canned, solids and liquids								
1 cup, sliced (104g)	28	9	1	5	1	0	1738	3.1
Peppers, jalapeno, raw								
1 pepper (14g)	4	1	0	1	0	0	0	0.4
Peppers, sweet, green, boiled, drained, without salt								
1 tablespoon (12g)	3	0	0	1	0	0	0	0.1

Food Serving size	Cal.	Fat cal.	Prot.	Carb.	Fat	Chol.	Sod.	Fiber
Peppers, sweet, green, canned, solids and liquids								
1 cup, halves (140g)	25	0	1	6	0	0	1917	1.4
Peppers, sweet, green, raw								
1 cup, sliced (92g)	25	0	1	6	0	0	2	1.8
Peppers, sweet, yellow, raw								
10 strips (52g)	14	0	1	3	0	0	1	0.5
Pickle relish, hamburger								
1 tablespoon (15g)	19	1	0	5	0	0	164	0.4
Pickle relish, hot dog								
1 tablespoon (15g)	14	0	0	3	0	0	164	0.3
Pickle relish, sweet								
1 tablespoon (15g)	20	0	0	5	0	0	122	0.2
Pickle, cucumber, sour 1 large (4″ long) (135g)	15	0	0	3	0	0	1631	1.4
Pickle, cucumber, sweet								
1 cup, chopped (160g)	187	0	0	51	0	0	1502	1.6
Pickles, cucumber, dill 1 cup, chopped or diced (143g)	26	0	1	6	0	0	1833	1.4
Pimento, canned								
1 tablespoon (12g)	3	0	0	1	0	0	2	0.2
Poi								
1 cup (240g)	269	0	0	65	0	0	29	0.0
Potato pancakes, home-prepared								
1 pancake (76g)	207	95	5	22	11	73	386	1.5
Potato puffs, frozen, prepared								
1 puff (7g)	16	6	0	2	1	0	52	0.2
Potato salad								
1 cup (250g)	358		8	28	20	170	1323	2.5
Potatoes, au gratin, dry mix, prepared with water, whole milk and butter Yield, $\frac{1}{6}$ of 5.5 oz package (137g)	127	0	3	18	5	21	601	1.4

Food Serving size	Cal.	Fat cal.	Prot.	Carb.	Fat	Chol.	Sod.	Fiber
Potatoes, au gratin, home-prepared from recipe using butter								
1 cup (245g)	323	0	12	27	20	56	1061	4.9
Potatoes, baked, flesh and skin, without salt								
1 potato ($2\frac{1}{3}''$ × $4\frac{3}{4}''$)								
(202g)	220	0	4	51	0	0	16	4.0
Potatoes, baked, flesh, without salt								
$\frac{1}{2}$ cup (61g)	57	0	1	13	0	0	3	1.2
Potatoes, baked, skin, without salt								
1 potato skin (58g)	115	0	2	27	0	0	12	4.6
Potatoes, boiled, cooked in skin, flesh, without salt								
$\frac{1}{2}$ cup (78g)	68	0	2	16	0	0	3	1.6
Potatoes, boiled, cooked in skin, skin, without salt								
1 potato skin (34g)	27	0	1	6	Ü	0	5	1.0
Potatoes, boiled, cooked without skin, flesh, without salt								
$\frac{1}{2}$ cup (78g)	67	0	2	16	0	0	4	1.6
Potatoes, canned, drained solids								
1 potato (35g)	21	0	0	5	0	0	77	0.7
Potatoes, French fried, frozen, home-prepared, heated in oven, without salt								
10 strips (50g)	100	35	2	16	4	0	15	1.5
Potatoes, French fried, frozen, par fried, cottage-cut, prepared, heated in oven, without salt								
10 strips (50g)	109	35	2	17	4	0	23	1.5
Potatoes, frozen, whole, boiled, drained, without salt								
100 grams	65	0	2	15	0	0	20	1.0
Potatoes, hashed brown, frozen, plain, prepared								
1 oval patty (approx $3''$ × $1\frac{1}{2}''$ × $\frac{1}{2}''$)	63	29	1	8	3	0	10	0.6
Potatoes, hashed brown, home-prepared								
1 cup (156g)	326	183	3	33	22	0	37	3.1
Potatoes, mashed, dehydrated, prepared from flakes without milk, whole milk and butter added								
1 cup (210g)	237	105	4	32	13	29	697	4.2

Food Serving size	Cal.	Fat cal.	Prot.	Carb.	Fat	Chol.	Sod.	Fiber
Potatoes, mashed, dehydrated, prepared from granules with milk, water and margarine added								
1 cup (210g)	166	37	4	27	4	4	491	4.2
Potatoes, mashed, home-prepared, whole milk and margarine added								
1 cup (210g)	223	74	4	36	8	4	620	4.2
Potatoes, microwaved, cooked in skin, flesh and skin, without salt								
1 potato, ($2\frac{1}{2}''$ dia.)								
(202g)	212	0	4	48	0	0	16	4.0
Potatoes, O'Brien, frozen, prepared								
100 grams	204	109	2	22	13	0	43	2.0
Potatoes, O'Brien, home-prepared								
1 cup (194g)	157	16	4	29	2	8	421	
Potatoes, scalloped, dry mix, prepared with water, whole milk and butter								
Yield, $\frac{1}{6}$ of 5.5 oz								
package (137g)	127	46	3	18	5	15	467	1.4
Potatoes, scalloped, home-prepared with butter								
1 cup (245g)	211	0	7	27	10	29	821	4.9
Pumpkin pie mix, canned								
1 cup (270g)	281	0	3	70	0	0	562	21.6
Pumpkin, boiled, drained, without salt								
1 cup, mashed (245g)	49	0	2	12	0	0	2	2.5
Pumpkin, canned, without salt								
1 cup (245g)	83	0	2	20	0	0	12	7.3
Radicchio, raw								
1 leaf (8g)	2	0	0	0	0	0	2	0.1
Radishes, raw								
1 large ($1''$ to $1\frac{1}{4}''$ dia)								
(9g)	2	1	0	0	0	0	2	0.2
Rutabagas, boiled, drained, without salt								
1 cup, cubes (170g)	66	0	2	15	0	0	34	3.4
Salsify, boiled, drained, without salt								
1 cup, sliced (135g)	92	0	4	20	0	0	22	4.1
Sauerkraut, canned, solids and liquids								
1 cup (142g)	27	0	1	6	0	0	939	2.8

Food Serving size	Cal.	Fat cal.	Prot.	Carb.	Fat	Chol.	Sod.	Fiber
Seaweed, kelp, raw $\frac{1}{8}$ cup or 2 tablespoons (10g)	4	1	0	1	0	0	23	0.1
Shallots, raw 1 tablespoon, chopped (10g)	7	0	0	2	0	0	1	
Soybeans, green, boiled, drained, without salt 1 cup (180g)	254	90	22	20	11	0	25	7.2
Soybeans, mature seeds, sprouted, steamed 1 cup (94g)	76	31	8	7	4	0	9	0.9
Soybeans, mature seeds, sprouted, stir-fried 100 grams	125	59	13	9	7	0	14	1.0
Spinach souffle 1 cup (136g)	219	0	11	3	19	184	763	
Spinach, boiled, drained, without salt 1 cup (180g)	41	0	5	7	0	0	126	3.6
Spinach, canned, drained solids 1 cup (214g)	49	0	6	6	0	0	58	4.3
Spinach, frozen, chopped or leaf, boiled, drained, without salt $\frac{1}{2}$ cup (95g)	27	0	3	5	0	0	82	2.8
Spinach, raw 1 cup (30g)	7	0	1	1	0	0	24	0.9
Squash, summer, all varieties, boiled, drained, without salt 1 cup, sliced (180g)	36	0	2	7	0	0	2	1.8
Squash, summer, all varieties, raw 1 cup, sliced (113g)	23	0	1	5	0	0	2	2.3
Squash, summer, crookneck and straightneck, boiled, drained, without salt $\frac{1}{2}$ cup slices (90g)	18	0	1	4	0	0	1	0.9
Squash, summer, crookneck and straightneck, canned, drained, solid, without salt 1 cup, diced (210g)	27	0	2	6	0	0	11	2.1
Squash, summer, crookneck and straightneck, raw 1 cup, sliced (130g)	25	0	1	5	0	0	3	2.6

Food Serving size	Cal.	Fat cal.	Prot.	Carb.	Fat	Chol.	Sod.	Fiber
Squash, summer, scallop, boiled, drained, without salt								
1 cup, sliced (180g)	29	0	2	5	0	0	2	3.6
Squash, summer, scallop, raw								
1 cup, slices (130g)	23	0	1	5	0	0	1	
Squash, summer, zucchini, includes skin, boiled, drained, without salt								
$\frac{1}{2}$ cup mashed (120g)	19	0	1	5	0	0	4	1.2
Squash, summer, zucchini, includes skin, raw								
1 cup, sliced (113g)	16	0	1	3	0	0	3	1.1
Squash, summer, zucchini, Italian style, canned								
1 cup (227g)	66	0	2	16	0	0	849	
Squash, winter, acorn, baked, without salt								
1 cup, cubes (205g)	115	0	2	31	0	0	8	8.2
Squash, winter, acorn, boiled, mashed, without salt								
1 cup, mashed (245g)	83	0	2	22	0	0	7	7.3
Squash, winter, acorn, raw								
1 cup, cubes (140g)	56	0	1	14	0	0	4	2.8
Squash, winter, all varieties, baked, without salt								
1 cup, cubes (205g)	80	17	2	18	2	0	2	6.2
Squash, winter, all varieties, raw								
1 cup, cubes (116g)	43	0	1	10	0	0	5	2.3
Squash, winter, butternut, baked, without salt								
1 cup, cubes (205g)	82	0	2	21	0	0	8	
Squash, winter, butternut, raw								
1 cup, cubes (140g)	63	0	1	17	0	0	6	
Squash, winter, hubbard, baked, without salt								
1 cup, cubes (205g)	103	17	4	23	2	0	16	
Squash, winter, hubbard, boiled, mashed, without salt								
1 cup, mashed (236g)	71	0	2	14	0	0	12	7.1
Squash, winter, hubbard, raw								
1 cup, cubes (116g)	46	0	2	10	0	0	8	
Squash, winter, spaghetti, boiled, drained, or baked, without salt								
1 cup (155g)	42	0	2	9	0	0	28	1.5
Squash, winter, spaghetti, raw								
1 cup, cubes (101g)	31	8	1	7	1	0	17	

Food Serving size	Cal.	Fat cal.	Prot.	Carb.	Fat	Chol.	Sod.	Fiber
Squash, zucchini, baby, raw 1 medium (11g)	2	0	0	0	0	0	0	0.1
Succotash (corn and limas), boiled, drained, without salt 1 cup (192g)	221	16	10	46	2	0	33	7.7
Succotash (corn and limas), canned, with cream style corn 1 cup (266g)	205	22	8	48	3	0	652	8.0
Succotash (corn and limas), canned, with whole kernel corn, solids and liquids 1 cup (255g)	161	0	8	36	0	0	564	7.7
Sweet potato, baked in skin, without salt 1 large (180g)	185	0	4	43	0	0	18	5.4
Sweet potato, boiled, without skin, without salt 1 medium (151g)	159	0	3	36	0	0	20	3.0
Sweet potato, canned, mashed 1 cup (255g)	258	0	5	59	0	0	191	5.1
Sweet potato, canned, syrup pack, drained solids 1 cup (196g)	212	0	2	49	0	0	76	5.9
Sweet potato, cooked, candied 1 piece ($2\frac{1}{2}$″ x 2″ dia) (105g)	144	0	1	29	3	8	74	2.1
Taro, tahitian, without salt 1 cup, slices (137g)	60	11	5	10	1	0	74	
Tomatillos, raw 1 medium (34g)	11	3	0	2	0	0	0	0.7
Tomato juice, canned, with salt added 6 fl oz (182g)	31	0	2	7	0	0	657	0.0
Tomato products, canned, paste, without salt added 1 tablespoon (16g)	13	1	1	3	0	0	14	0.6
Tomato products, canned, puree, without salt added 1 cup (250g)	100	0	5	25	0	0	85	5.0
Tomato products, canned, sauce, Spanish style 1 cup (244g)	81	0	2	17	0	0	1152	2.4
Tomato products, canned, sauce, with herbs and cheese $\frac{1}{2}$ cup (122g)	72	21	2	12	2	4	662	2.4

Food Serving size	Cal.	Fat cal.	Prot.	Carb.	Fat	Chol.	Sod.	Fiber
Tomato products, canned, sauce, with mushrooms 1 cup (245g)	86	0	2	20	0	0	1107	4.9
Tomato products, canned, sauce, with onions, green peppers, and celery 1 cup (250g)	103	21	3	23	3	0	1365	2.5
Tomato products, canned, sauce, with onions 1 cup (245g)	103	0	5	25	0	0	1350	4.9
Tomato products, canned, sauce 1 cup (245g)	74	0	2	17	0	0	1482	2.5
Tomatoes, green, raw 1 cup (180g)	43	0	2	9	0	0	23	1.8
Tomatoes, red, ripe, boiled, without salt 1 cup (240g)	65	0	2	14	0	0	26	2.4
Tomatoes, red, ripe, stewed 1 cup (101g)	80		2	13	3	0	460	2.0
Tomatoes, red, ripe, canned, stewed 1 cup (255g)	71	0	3	18	0	0	564	2.5
Tomatoes, red, ripe, canned, whole, regular pack 1 tablespoon (15g)	3	0	0	1	0	0	22	0.2
Tomatoes, red, ripe, raw, year round average 1 cup, cherry tomato (149g)	31	0	1	7	0	0	13	1.5
Tomatoes, sun-dried, packed in oil, drained 1 piece (3g)	6	4	0	1	0	0	8	0.2
Tomatoes, sun-dried 1 piece (2g)	5	1	0	1	0	0	42	0.2
Turnip greens, boiled, drained, without salt 1 cup, chopped (144g)	29	0	1	6	0	0	42	5.8
Turnip greens, canned, solids and liquids $\frac{1}{2}$ cup (117g)	16	0	1	2	0	0	324	2.3
Turnips, boiled, drained, without salt 1 cup, cubes (156g)	33	0	2	8	0	0	78	3.1
Vegetable juice cocktail, canned 6 fl oz (182g)	35	0	2	9	0	0	491	1.8

Food Serving size	Cal.	Fat cal.	Prot.	Carb.	Fat	Chol.	Sod.	Fiber
Vegetables, mixed, canned, drained solids								
1 cup (163g)	77	0	5	15	0	0	243	4.9
Vegetables, mixed, frozen, boiled, drained, without salt								
$\frac{1}{2}$ cup (91g)	54	0	3	12	0	0	32	3.6
Water chestnuts, Chinese, canned, solids and liquids								
4 waterchestnuts (28g)	14	0	0	3	0	0	2	0.6
Watercress, raw								
1 sprig (2g)	0	0	0	0	0	0	1	0.0
Waxgourd, (Chinese preserving melon), boiled, drained, without salt								
1 cup, cubes (175g)	23	0	0	5	0	0	187	1.8
Yam, boiled or baked, drained, without salt								
$\frac{1}{2}$ cup cubes (68g)	79	0	1	19	0	0	5	2.7
Yam, raw								
1 cup, cubes (150g)	177	0	3	42	0	0	14	6.0
Yambean (jicama), boiled, drained, without salt								
100 grams	38	0	1	9	0	0	4	
Yambean (jicama), raw								
1 cup, slices (120g)	46	0	1	11	0	0	5	6.0
Yardlong bean, boiled, drained, without salt								
1 pod (14g)	7	0	0	1	0	0	1	

Legumes and Legume Products

Food Serving size	Cal.	Fat cal.	Prot.	Carb.	Fat	Chol.	Sod.	Fiber
Beans								
Beans, adzuki, mature seed, boiled, with salt 1 cup (230g)	294	0	18	58	0	0	561	
Beans, adzuki, mature seeds, boiled, without salt 1 cup (230g)	294	0	18	58	0	0	18	
Beans, adzuki, mature seeds, canned, sweetened 1 cup (296g)	702	0	12	163	0	0	645	
Beans, baked, canned, plain or vegetarian 1 cup (254g)	236	0	13	53	0	0	1008	12.7
Beans, baked, canned, with beef 1 cup (266g)	322	72	16	45	8	59	1264	
Beans, baked, canned, with franks 1 cup (259g)	368	163	18	39	18	16	1114	18.1
Beans, baked, canned, with pork and sweet sauce 1 cup (253g)	281	23	13	53	3	18	850	12.6
Beans, baked, canned, with pork and tomato sauce 1 tablespoon (16g)	16	1	1	3	0	1	70	0.8
Beans, baked, canned, with pork 1 cup (253g)	268	45	13	51	5	18	1047	15.2
Beans, baked, home prepared 1 cup (253g)	382	111	15	53	13	13	1068	15.2

Food Serving size	Cal.	Fat cal.	Prot.	Carb.	Fat	Chol.	Sod.	Fiber
Beans, black turtle soup, mature seeds, boiled, with salt								
1 cup (185g)	241	0	15	44	0	0	442	9.3
Beans, black turtle soup, mature seeds, boiled, without salt								
1 cup (185g)	241	0	15	44	0	0	6	9.3
Beans, black turtle soup, mature seeds, canned								
1 cup (240g)	218	0	14	41	0	0	922	16.8
Beans, black, mature seeds, boiled, with salt								
1 cup (172g)	227	14	15	41	2	0	408	15.5
Beans, black, mature seeds, boiled, without salt								
1 cup (172g)	227	14	15	41	2	0	2	15.5
Beans, cranberry (roman), mature seeds, raw								
1 cup (195g)	653	16	45	117	2	0	12	48.8
Beans, fava, in pod, raw								
1 pod (6g)	5	1	0	1	0	0	2	
Beans, French, mature seeds, boiled, with salt								
1 cup (177g)	228	15	12	42	2	0	428	15.9
Beans, French, mature seeds, boiled, without salt								
1 cup (177g)	228	15	12	42	2	0	11	15.9
Beans, great northern, mature seeds, boiled, with salt								
1 cup (177g)	209	0	14	37	0	0	421	12.4
Beans, great northern, mature seeds, boiled, without salt								
1 cup (177g)	209	0	14	37	0	0	4	12.4
Beans, great northern, mature seeds, canned								
1 cup (262g)	299	0	18	55	0	0	10	13.1
Beans, kidney, all types, mature seeds, boiled, with salt								
1 cup (177g)	225	0	16	41	0	0	421	10.6
Beans, kidney, all types, mature seeds, boiled, without salt								
1 tablespoon (11g)	14	0	1	3	0	0	0	0.7
Beans, kidney, all types, mature seeds, canned								
1 cup (256g)	207	0	13	38	0	0	888	10.2
Beans, kidney, California red, mature seeds, boiled, with salt								
1 cup (177g)	219	0	16	39	0	0	425	15.9
Beans, kidney, California red, mature seeds, boiled, without salt								
1 cup (177g)	219	0	16	39	0	0	7	15.9

Food Serving size	Cal.	Fat cal.	Prot.	Carb.	Fat	Chol.	Sod.	Fiber
Beans, kidney, mature seeds, sprouted, boiled, drained, without salt								
100 grams	33	8	5	5	1	0	7	
Beans, kidney, red, mature seeds, boiled, with salt								
1 cup (177g)	225	0	16	41	0	0	421	12.4
Beans, kidney, red, mature seeds, boiled, without salt								
1 tablespoon (11g)	14	0	1	3	0	0	0	0.8
Beans, kidney, red, mature seeds, canned								
1 tablespoon (16g)	14	0	1	3	0	0	55	1.0
Beans, kidney, royal red, mature seeds, boiled with salt								
1 cup (177g)	218	0	16	39	0	0	427	15.9
Beans, kidney, royal red, mature seeds, boiled, without salt								
1 cup (177g)	218	0	16	39	0	0	9	15.9
Beans, lima, immature seeds, boiled, drained, without salt								
1 cup (170g)	209	0	12	41	0	0	29	8.5
Beans, lima, immature seeds, canned, regular pack, solids and liquids								
½ cup (124g)	88	0	5	16	0	0	312	5.0
Beans, lima, large, mature seeds, boiled, with salt								
1 cup (188g)	216	0	15	39	0	0	447	13.2
Beans, lima, large, mature seeds, boiled, without salt								
1 tablespoon (12g)	14	0	1	3	0	0	0	0.8
Beans, lima, large, mature seeds, canned								
1 cup (241g)	190	0	12	36	0	0	810	12.1
Beans, lima, thin seeded (baby), mature seeds, boiled, with salt								
1 cup (182g)	229	0	15	42	0	0	435	14.6
Beans, lima, thin seeded (baby), mature seeds, boiled, without salt								
1 cup (182g)	229	0	15	42	0	0	5	14.6
Beans, mung, mature seeds, boiled, with salt								
1 cup (202g)	212	0	14	38	0	0	481	16.2
Beans, mung, mature seeds, boiled, without salt								
1 cup (202g)	212	0	14	38	0	0	4	16.2
Beans, mung, mature seeds, sprouted, boiled, drained, without salt								
1 cup (124g)	26	0	2	5	0	0	12	1.2
Beans, mung, mature seeds, sprouted, stir-fried								
1 cup (124g)	62	0	5	14	0	0	11	2.5

Food
Serving size

	Cal.	Fat cal.	Prot.	Carb.	Fat	Chol.	Sod.	Fiber
Beans, mung, mature seeds, sprouted, canned, drained solids								
1 cup (125g)	15	0	1	3	0	0	175	1.3
Beans, mungo, mature seeds, boiled, with salt								
1 cup (180g)	189	15	14	32	2	0	437	10.8
Beans, mungo, mature seeds, boiled, without salt								
1 oz dry, yield after cooking (69g)	72	6	6	12	1	0	5	4.1
Beans, navy, mature seeds, boiled, with salt								
1 cup (182g)	258	15	16	47	2	0	431	10.9
Beans, navy, mature seeds, boiled, without salt								
1 cup (182g)	258	15	16	47	2	0	2	10.9
Beans, navy, mature seeds, canned								
1 cup (262g)	296	0	21	52	0	0	1174	13.1
Beans, navy, mature seeds, sprouted, boiled, drained, without salt								
100 grams	78	8	7	15	1	0	14	
Beans, pink, mature seeds, boiled, with salt								
1 cup (169g)	252	0	15	47	0	0	402	8.4
Beans, pink, mature seeds, boiled, without salt								
1 cup (169g)	252	0	15	47	0	0	3	8.4
Beans, pinto, immature seeds, frozen, boiled, drained, without salt								
yield, $\frac{1}{3}$ of 10 oz package (94g)	152	0	8	29	0	0	78	8.5
Beans, pinto, mature seeds, boiled, with salt								
1 cup (171g)	234	14	14	44	2	0	407	15.4
Beans, pinto, mature seeds, boiled, without salt								
1 tablespoon (11g)	15	1	1	3	0	0	0	1.0
Beans, pinto, mature seeds, canned								
1 cup (240g)	206	20	12	36	2	0	706	12.0
Beans, refried, canned								
1 tablespoon (16g)	15	1	1	3	0	1	48	0.8
Beans, shell, canned, solids and liquids								
1 cup (245g)	74	0	5	15	0	0	818	7.3
Beans, small white, mature seeds, boiled, with salt								
1 cup (179g)	254	15	16	47	2	0	426	17.9

Food Serving size	Cal.	Fat cal.	Prot.	Carb.	Fat	Chol.	Sod.	Fiber
Beans, small white, mature seeds, boiled, without salt								
1 cup (179g)	254	15	16	47	2	0	4	17.9
Beans, snap, canned, all styles, seasoned, solids and liquids								
$\frac{1}{2}$ cup (114g)	18	0	1	3	0	0	425	2.3
Beans, snap, green, boiled, drained, without salt								
1 cup (125g)	44	0	3	10	0	0	4	3.8
Beans, snap, green, frozen, boiled, drained without salt								
1 cup (135g)	38	0	1	8	0	0	12	4.1
Beans, soy, mature seeds, boiled, with salt								
1 cup (172g)	298	130	29	17	15	0	408	10.3
Beans, soy, mature seeds, boiled, without salt								
1 tablespoon (11g)	19	8	2	1	1	0	0	0.7
Beans, soy, mature seeds, dry roasted								
1 cup (172g)	774	317	69	57	38	0	3	13.8
Beans, soy, mature seeds, roasted, no salt added								
1 cup (172g)	810	360	60	58	43	0	7	31.0
Beans, soy, mature seeds, roasted, salted								
1 cup (172g)	810	360	60	58	43	0	280	31.0
Beans, white, mature seeds, boiled, with salt								
1 cup (179g)	249	0	18	45	0	0	433	10.7
Beans, white, mature seeds, boiled, without salt								
1 tablespoon (11g)	15	0	1	3	0	0	1	0.7
Beans, white, mature seeds, canned								
1 cup (262g)	307	0	18	58	0	0	13	13.1
Beans, winged, mature seeds, boiled, without salt								
1 cup (172g)	253	86	19	26	10	0	22	
Beans, winged, mature seeds, boiled, with salt								
1 cup (172g)	253	86	19	26	10	0	428	
Beans, yardlong, mature seeds, boiled, without salt								
1 cup (171g)	202	0	14	36	0	0	9	6.8
Beans, yardlong, yardlong, mature seeds, boiled, with salt								
1 cup (171g)	202	0	14	36	0	0	412	6.8
Beans, yellow, mature seeds, boiled, with salt								
1 cup (177g)	255	15	16	44	2	0	427	17.7

Food Serving size	Cal.	Fat cal.	Prot.	Carb.	Fat	Chol.	Sod.	Fiber
Beans, yellow, mature seeds, boiled, without salt								
1 cup (177g)	255	15	16	44	2	0	9	17.7
Broadbeans (fava beans), mature seeds, boiled, with salt								
1 cup (170g)	187	0	14	34	0	0	410	8.5
Broadbeans (fava beans), mature seeds, boiled, without salt								
1 cup (170g)	187	0	14	34	0	0	9	8.5
Broadbeans (fava beans), mature seeds, canned								
1 cup (256g)	182	0	13	31	0	0	1160	10.2
Chickpeas (garbanzo beans, bengal gram), mature seeds, boiled, with salt								
1 cup (164g)	269	41	15	44	5	0	399	13.1
Chickpeas (garbanzo beans, bengal gram), mature seeds, boiled, without salt								
1 cup (164g)	269	41	15	44	5	0	11	13.1
Chickpeas (garbanzo beans, bengal gram), mature seeds, canned								
1 cup (240g)	286	20	12	55	2	0	718	9.6
Chili with beans, canned								
1 tablespoon (16g)	18	7	1	2	1	3	84	0.6
Cowpeas (Blackeyes), immature seeds, boiled, drained, without salt								
1 cup (165g)	160	0	5	33	0	0	7	8.3
Cowpeas, catjang, mature seeds, boiled, with salt								
1 cup (171g)	200	14	14	34	2	0	436	6.8
Cowpeas, catjang, mature seeds, boiled, without salt								
1 cup (171g)	200	14	14	34	2	0	32	6.8
Cowpeas, common (blackeyes, crowder, southern), mature seeds, boiled, with salt								
1 cup (171g)	198	14	14	36	2	0	410	10.3
Cowpeas, common (blackeyes, crowder, southern), mature seeds, boiled, without salt								
1 cup (172g)	200	14	14	36	2	0	7	10.3
Cowpeas, common (blackeyes, crowder, southern), mature seeds, canned with pork								
1 cup (240g)	199		7	41	5	17	840	7.2

Food Serving size	Cal.	Fat cal.	Prot.	Carb.	Fat	Chol.	Sod.	Fiber
Cowpeas, common (blackeyes, crowder, southern), mature seeds, canned, plain								
1 cup (240g)	185	20	12	34	2	0	718	7.2
Cowpeas, leafy tips, boiled, drained, without salt								
1 cup, chopped (53g)	12	0	3	2	0	0	3	
Cowpeas, young pods with seeds, boiled, drained, without salt								
1 cup (95g)	32	0	3	7	0	0	3	
Hyacinth beans, mature seeds, boiled, without salt								
1 cup (194g)	227	16	16	41	2	0	14	
Lentils, mature seeds, boiled, with salt								
1 cup (198g)	230	0	18	40	0	0	471	15.8
Lentils, mature seeds, boiled, without salt								
1 tablespoon (12g)	14	0	1	2	0	0	0	1.0
Lentils, pink, raw								
1 cup (192g)	664	32	48	113	4	0	13	21.1
Lupins, mature seeds, boiled, with salt								
1 cup (166g)	198	42	27	17	5	0	398	5.0
Lupins, mature seeds, boiled, without salt								
1 cup (166g)	198	42	27	17	5	0	7	5.0
Mothbeans, mature seeds, boiled, without salt								
1 cup (177g)	207	15	14	37	2	0	18	
Peas, split, mature seeds, boiled, with salt								
1 cup (196g)	231	0	16	41	0	0	466	15.7
Peas, split, mature seeds, boiled, without salt								
1 tablespoon (12g)	14	0	1	3	0	0	0	1.0
Pigeon peas (red gram), mature seeds, boiled, without salt								
1 cup (168g)	203	0	12	39	0	0	8	11.8

Peanuts

Food Serving size	Cal.	Fat cal.	Prot.	Carb.	Fat	Chol.	Sod.	Fiber
Peanut butter, chunk style, with salt								
2 tablespoons (32g)	188	134	8	7	16	0	156	2.2
Peanut butter, chunk style, without salt								
2 tablespoons (32g)	188	134	8	7	16	0	5	2.2
Peanut butter, smooth style, with salt								
2 tablespoons (32g)	190	137	8	6	16	0	149	1.9

Food Serving size	Cal.	Fat cal.	Prot.	Carb.	Fat	Chol.	Sod.	Fiber
Peanut butter, smooth style, without salt 2 tablespoons (32g)	190	137	8	6	16	0	5	1.9
Peanuts, all types, boiled, with salt 1 cup, in shell, edible yield (63g)	200	116	9	13	14	0	473	5.7
Peanuts, all types, dry-roasted, with salt 1 peanut (1g)	6	4	0	0	1	0	8	0.1
Peanuts, all types, dry-roasted, without salt 1 oz (28g)	164	117	7	6	14	0	2	2.2
Peanuts, all types, oil-roasted, with salt 1 cup, chopped (144g)	837	591	37	27	71	0	624	13.0
Peanuts, all types, oil-roasted, without salt 1 oz, shelled (28g)	163	115	7	5	14	0	2	2.0
Peanuts, all types, raw 1 oz (28g)	159	115	7	4	14	0	5	2.2
Peanuts, Spanish, oil-roasted, with salt 1 oz (28g)	162	115	8	5	14	0	121	2.5
Peanuts, Spanish, oil-roasted, without salt 1 oz (28g)	162	115	8	5	14	0	2	2.5
Peanuts, Spanish, raw 1 oz (28g)	160	117	7	4	14	0	6	2.8
Peanuts, Valencia, oil-roasted, with salt 1 oz (28g)	165	120	8	4	14	0	216	2.5
Peanuts, Valencia, oil-roasted, without salt 1 oz (28g)	165	120	8	4	14	0	2	2.5
Peanuts, Valencia, raw 1 oz (28g)	160	112	7	6	13	0	0	2.5
Peanuts, Virginia, oil-roasted, with salt 1 oz (28g)	162	115	7	6	14	0	121	2.5
Peanuts, Virginia, oil-roasted, without salt 1 oz (28g)	162	115	7	6	14	0	2	2.5
Peanuts, Virginia, raw 1 oz (28g)	158	115	7	5	14	0	3	2.2

Food Serving size	Cal.	Fat cal.	Prot.	Carb.	Fat	Chol.	Sod.	Fiber

Legume Products

Bacon, meatless
1 oz, raw (yield
after cooking) (16g) | 50 | 40 | 2 | 1 | 5 | 0 | 234 | 0.5

Falafel
1 patty (approx
$2\frac{1}{4}''$ dia) (17g) | 57 | 0 | 2 | 5 | 3 | 0 | 50 |

Hummus, commercial
1 tablespoon (14g) | 23 | 12 | 1 | 2 | 1 | 0 | 53 | 0.8

Hummus, raw
1 tablespoon (15g) | 26 | 0 | 1 | 3 | 1 | 0 | 37 | 0.8

Meat extender
1 oz (28g) | 88 | 7 | 11 | 11 | 1 | 0 | 3 | 5.0

Miso
1 cup (275g) | 567 | 138 | 33 | 77 | 17 | 0 | 10029 | 13.8

Natto
1 cup (175g) | 371 | 161 | 32 | 25 | 19 | 0 | 12 | 8.8

Sausage, meatless
1 link (25g) | 64 | 38 | 5 | 3 | 5 | 0 | 222 | 0.8

Soy milk, fluid
1 fl oz (31g) | 10 | 5 | 1 | 1 | 1 | 0 | 4 | 0.3

Soy protein concentrate, produced by alcohol extraction
1 oz (28g) | 93 | 0 | 16 | 9 | 0 | 0 | 1 | 1.7

Soy protein isolate
1 oz (28g) | 95 | 7 | 23 | 2 | 1 | 0 | 281 | 1.7

Soy sauce made from hydrolyzed vegetable protein
1 teaspoon (6g) | 2 | 0 | 0 | 0 | 0 | 0 | 341 | 0.0

Soy sauce made from soy (tamari)
1 teaspoon (6g) | 4 | 0 | 1 | 0 | 0 | 0 | 335 | 0.1

Soy sauce made from soy and wheat (shoyu)
1 tablespoon (16g) | 8 | 0 | 1 | 1 | 0 | 0 | 914 | 0.2

Soy sauce made from soy and wheat (shoyu), low sodium
1 tablespoon (18g) | 10 | 0 | 1 | 2 | 0 | 0 | 600 | 0.2

Food Serving size	Cal.	Fat cal.	Prot.	Carb.	Fat	Chol.	Sod.	Fiber
Tempeh 1 cup (166g)	330	111	32	28	13	0	10	
Tofu, dried-frozen (koyadofu), prepared with calcium sulfate 1 piece (17g)	82	43	8	3	5	0	1	0.2
Tofu, dried-frozen (koyadofu) 1 piece (17g)	82	43	8	3	5	0	1	1.2
Tofu, fried, prepared with calcium sulfate 1 piece (13g)	35	22	2	1	3	0	2	0.5
Tofu, fried 1 piece (13g)	35	22	2	1	3	0	2	0.5
Tofu, okara 1 cup (122g)	94	20	4	16	2	0	11	
Tofu, raw, firm, prepared with calcium sulfate $\frac{1}{4}$ block (81g)	117	61	13	3	7	0	11	1.6
Tofu, raw, firm $\frac{1}{4}$ block (81g)	117	61	13	3	7	0	11	1.6
Tofu, raw, regular, prepared with calcium sulfate $\frac{1}{4}$ block (116g)	88	49	9	2	6	0	8	0.0
Tofu, raw, regular 1 cubic inch (18g)	14	8	1	0	1	0	1	0.2
Tofu, salted and fermented (fuyu), prepared with calcium sulfate 1 block (11g)	13	7	1	1	1	0	316	
Tofu, salted and fermented (fuyu) 1 block (11g)	13	7	1	1	1	0	316	

Fruits and Fruit Juices

Food Serving size	Cal.	Fat cal.	Prot.	Carb.	Fat	Chol.	Sod.	Fiber

Fruits

Apples, canned, sweetened, sliced, drained, unheated
| 1 cup, slices (204g) | 137 | 0 | 0 | 35 | 0 | 0 | 6 | 4.1 |

Apples, raw, with skin
| 1 cup, slices (110g) | 65 | 0 | 0 | 17 | 0 | 0 | 0 | 3.3 |

Apples, raw, without skin, cooked, boiled
| 1 cup, slices (171g) | 91 | 0 | 0 | 24 | 0 | 0 | 2 | 3.4 |

Apples, raw, without skin, cooked, microwave
| 1 cup, slices (170g) | 95 | 0 | 0 | 24 | 0 | 0 | 2 | 5.1 |

Apples, raw, without skin
| 1 cup, slices (110g) | 63 | 0 | 0 | 17 | 0 | 0 | 0 | 2.2 |

Applesauce, canned, sweetened, without salt
| 1 cup, sauce (255g) | 194 | 0 | 0 | 51 | 0 | 0 | 8 | 2.5 |

Applesauce, canned, unsweetened, without added ascorbic acid
| 1 cup (244g) | 105 | 0 | 0 | 27 | 0 | 0 | 5 | 2.4 |

Apricot nectar, canned, without added ascorbic acid
| 1 fl oz (31g) | 17 | 0 | 0 | 4 | 0 | 0 | 1 | 0.3 |

Apricots, canned, extra heavy syrup pack, without skin, solids and liquids
| 1 cup whole, without
pits (246g) | 236 | 0 | 2 | 62 | 0 | 0 | 32 | 4.9 |

Food Serving size	Cal.	Fat cal.	Prot.	Carb.	Fat	Chol.	Sod.	Fiber
Apricots, canned, extra light syrup pack, with skin, solids and liquids								
1 cup, halves (247g)	121	0	2	30	0	0	5	4.9
Apricots, canned, heavy syrup pack, with skin, solids and liquids								
1 cup, whole (240g)	199	0	2	50	0	0	10	4.8
Apricots, canned, heavy syrup pack, without skin, solids and liquids								
1 cup whole, without pits (258g)	214	0	3	54	0	0	28	5.2
Apricots, canned, juice pack, with skin, solids and liquids								
1 apricot half with liquid (36g)	17	0	0	4	0	0	1	0.7
Apricots, canned, light syrup pack, with skin, solids and liquids								
1 apricot half with liquid (40g)	25	0	0	6	0	0	2	0.8
Apricots, canned, water pack, with skin, solids and liquids								
1 apricot half with liquid (36g)	10	0	0	2	0	0	1	0.7
Apricots, canned, water pack, without skin, solids and liquids								
1 cup whole, without pits (227g)	50	0	2	11	0	0	25	2.3
Apricots, dried, sulfured, stewed, with added sugar								
1 cup, halves (270g)	305	0	3	78	0	0	8	10.8
Apricots, dried, sulfured, stewed, without added sugar								
1 cup, halves (250g)	213	0	3	55	0	0	8	7.5
Apricots, dried, sulfured, uncooked								
1 half (4g)	10	0	0	2	0	0	0	0.4
Apricots, raw								
1 cup, halves (155g)	74	0	2	17	0	0	2	3.1
Avocados, raw, all commercial varieties								
1 cup, cubes (150g)	242	188	3	11	23	0	15	7.5
Avocados, raw, California								
1 fruit, without skin and seeds (173g)	306	246	3	12	29	0	21	8.6
Avocados, raw, Florida								
1 cup, pureed (230g)	258	173	5	21	21	0	12	11.5
Bananas, raw								
1 cup, sliced (150g)	138	0	2	35	0	0	2	3.0

Food Serving size	Cal.	Fat cal.	Prot.	Carb.	Fat	Chol.	Sod.	Fiber
Blackberries, canned, heavy syrup, solids and liquids								
1 cup (256g)	236	0	3	59	0	0	8	7.7
Blackberries, frozen, unsweetened								
1 cup (151g)	97	0	2	24	0	0	2	7.6
Blackberries, raw								
1 cup (144g)	75	0	1	19	0	0	0	7.2
Blueberries, canned, heavy syrup, solids and liquids								
1 cup (256g)	225	0	3	56	0	0	8	5.1
Blueberries, frozen, sweetened								
1 cup, thawed (230g)	186	0	0	51	0	0	2	4.6
Blueberries, frozen, unsweetened								
1 cup, unthawed (155g)	79	13	0	19	2	0	2	4.7
Blueberries, raw								
1 cup, unthawed (145g)	81	0	1	20	0	0	9	4.3
Boysenberries, canned, heavy syrup								
1 cup (256g)	225	0	3	56	0	0	8	7.7
Boysenberries, frozen, unsweetened								
1 cup (132g)	66	0	1	16	0	0	1	5.3
Breadfruit, raw								
$\frac{1}{4}$ small fruit (96g)	99	0	1	26	0	0	2	4.8
Cherries, sour, red, canned, extra heavy syrup pack, solids and liquids								
1 cup (261g)	298	0	3	76	0	0	18	2.6
Cherries, sour, red, canned, heavy syrup pack, solids and liquids								
1 cup (256g)	233	0	3	59	0	0	18	2.6
Cherries, sour, red, canned, light syrup pack, solids and liquids								
1 cup (252g)	189	0	3	48	0	0	18	2.5
Cherries, sour, red, canned, water pack, solids and liquids								
1 cup (244g)	88	0	2	22	0	0	17	2.4
Cherries, sour, red, raw								
1 cup with pits (103g)	52	0	1	12	0	0	3	2.1
Cherries, sweet, canned, extra heavy syrup pack, solids and liquids								
1 cup, pitted (261g)	266	0	3	68	0	0	8	5.2
Cherries, sweet, canned, heavy syrup pack, solids and liquids								
1 cup, pitted (253g)	210	0	3	53	0	0	8	5.1

Food Serving size	Cal.	Fat cal.	Prot.	Carb.	Fat	Chol.	Sod.	Fiber
Cherries, sweet, canned, juice pack, solids and liquids								
1 cup, pitted (250g)	135	0	3	35	0	0	8	5.0
Cherries, sweet, canned, light syrup pack, solids and liquids								
1 cup, pitted (252g)	169	0	3	43	0	0	8	5.0
Cherries, sweet, canned, water pack, solids and liquids								
1 cup, pitted (248g)	114	0	2	30	0	0	2	5.0
Cherries, sweet, raw								
1 cup, with pits, yields (117g)	84	10	1	20	1	0	0	2.3
Crabapples, raw								
1 cup, slices (110g)	84	0	0	22	0	0	1	
Cranberries, raw								
1 cup, whole (95g)	47	0	0	12	0	0	1	3.8
Cranberry sauce, canned, sweetened								
1 slice ($\frac{1}{2}''$ thick), approx 8 slices per can	86	0	0	22	0	0	17	0.6
Cranberry-orange relish, canned								
1 cup (275g)	490	0	0	127	0	0	88	0.0
Currants, European black, raw								
1 cup (112g)	71	0	1	17	0	0	2	
Currants, red and white, raw								
1 cup (112g)	63	0	1	16	0	0	1	4.5
Currants, zante, dried								
1 cup (144g)	408	0	6	107	0	0	12	10.1
Dates, domestic, natural and dry								
1 date (8g)	22	0	0	6	0	0	0	0.6
Elderberries, raw								
1 cup (145g)	106	0	1	26	0	0	9	10.1
Figs, canned, extra heavy syrup pack, solids and liquids								
1 cup (261g)	279	0	0	73	0	0	3	
Figs, canned, heavy syrup pack, solids and liquids								
1 fig with liquid (28g)	25	0	0	6	0	0	0	0.6
Figs, canned, light syrup pack, solids and liquids								
1 fig with liquid (28g)	19	0	0	5	0	0	0	0.6

Food Serving size	Cal.	Fat cal.	Prot.	Carb.	Fat	Chol.	Sod.	Fiber
Figs, canned, water pack, solids and liquids								
1 fig with liquid (27g)	14	0	0	4	0	0	0	0.5
Figs, dried, stewed								
1 cup (259g)	280	0	3	73	0	0	13	12.9
Figs, dried, uncooked								
1 fig (19g)	48	2	1	12	0	0	2	1.7
Figs, raw								
1 medium ($2\frac{1}{4}''$ dia)								
(50g)	37	0	1	10	0	0	1	1.5
Fruit cocktail (peach and pineapple and pear and grape and cherry), canned, extra heavy syrup, solids and liquids								
$\frac{1}{2}$ cup (130g)	114	0	0	30	0	0	8	1.3
Fruit cocktail (peach and pineapple and pear and grape and cherry), canned, extra light syrup, solids and liquids								
$\frac{1}{2}$ cup (123g)	55	0	0	15	0	0	5	1.2
Fruit cocktail (peach and pineapple and pear and grape and cherry), canned, heavy syrup, solids and liquids								
1 cup (248g)	181	0	0	47	0	0	15	2.5
Fruit cocktail (peach and pineapple and pear and grape and cherry), canned, juice pack, solids and liquids								
1 cup (237g)	109	0	0	28	0	0	9	2.4
Fruit cocktail (peach and pineapple and pear and grape and cherry), canned, light syrup, solids and liquids								
1 cup (242g)	138	0	0	36	0	0	15	2.4
Fruit cocktail (peach and pineapple and pear and grape and cherry), canned, water pack, solids and liquids								
1 cup (237g)	76	0	0	21	0	0	9	2.4
Fruit salad (peach and pear and apricot and pineapple and cherry), canned, extra heavy syrup, solids and liquids								
1 cup (259g)	228	0	0	60	0	0	13	2.6
Fruit salad (peach and pear and apricot and pineapple and cherry), canned, heavy syrup, solids and liquids								
1 cup (255g)	186	0	0	48	0	0	15	2.5
Fruit salad (peach and pear and apricot and pineapple and cherry), canned, juice pack, solids and liquids								
1 cup (249g)	125	0	2	32	0	0	12	2.5

Food Serving size	Cal.	Fat cal.	Prot.	Carb.	Fat	Chol.	Sod.	Fiber
Fruit salad (peach and pear and apricot and pineapple and cherry), canned, light syrup, solids and liquids								
1 cup (252g)	146	0	0	38	0	0	15	2.5
Fruit salad (peach and pear and apricot and pineapple and cherry), canned, water pack, solids and liquids								
1 cup (245g)	74	0	0	20	0	0	7	2.5
Fruit salad (pineapple and papaya and banana and guava), tropical, canned, heavy syrup, solids and liquids								
1 cup (257g)	221	0	0	57	0	0	5	2.6
Fruit, mixed (peach and pear and pineapple), canned, heavy syrup, solids and liquids								
1 cup (255g)	184	0	0	48	0	0	10	2.5
Gooseberries, canned, light syrup pack, solids and liquids								
1 cup (252g)	184	0	3	48	0	0	5	5.0
Gooseberries, raw								
1 cup (150g)	66	13	2	15	2	0	2	6.0
Grapefruit, raw, pink and red and white, all areas								
$\frac{1}{2}$ large fruit (approx $4\frac{1}{2}''$ dia) (166g)	53	0	2	13	0	0	0	1.7
Grapefruit, raw, pink and red, all areas								
$\frac{1}{2}$ fruit, ($3\frac{3}{4}''$ dia, sphere) (123g)	37	0	1	10	0	0	0	
Grapefruit, raw, white, all areas								
$\frac{1}{2}$ fruit, ($3\frac{3}{4}''$ dia, sphere) (118g)	39	0	1	9	0	0	0	1.2
Grapefruit, sections, canned, juice pack, solids and liquids								
1 cup (249g)	92	0	2	22	0	0	17	0.0
Grapefruit, sections, canned, light syrup pack, solids and liquids								
1 cup (254g)	152	0	3	38	0	0	5	0.0
Grapefruit, sections, canned, water pack, solids and liquids								
1 cup (244g)	88	0	2	22	0	0	5	0.0
Grapes, American type (slip skin), raw								
1 grape (2g)	1	0	0	0	0	0	0	0.0

Food Serving size	Cal.	Fat cal.	Prot.	Carb.	Fat	Chol.	Sod.	Fiber
Grapes, canned, Thompson seedless, heavy syrup pack, solids and liquids								
1 cup (256g)	187	0	0	51	0	0	13	0.0
Grapes, canned, Thompson seedless, water pack, solids and liquids								
1 cup (245g)	98	0	0	25	0	0	15	2.5
Grapes, European type (adherent skin), raw 1 cup, with seeds, yields (154g)	109	13	2	28	2	0	3	1.5
Guavas, common, raw 1 fruit, without refuse (90g)	46	8	1	11	1	0	3	4.5
Guavas, strawberry, raw 1 fruit, without refuse (6g)	4	1	0	1	0	0	2	
Kiwi fruit (Chinese gooseberries), fresh, raw 1 large fruit, without skin (91g)	56	0	1	14	0	0	5	2.7
Kumquats, raw 1 fruit, without refuse (19g)	12	0	0	3	0	0	1	1.3
Lemons, raw, without peel 1 fruit ($2\frac{1}{8}''$ dia) (58g)	17	0	1	5	0	0	1	1.7
Limes, raw 1 fruit (2″ dia) (67g)	20	0	1	7	0	0	1	2.0
Litchis, dried 1 nut (2g)	6	0	0	1	0	0	0	0.1
Litchis, raw 1 fruit, without refuse (10g)	7	0	0	2	0	0	0	0.1
Loganberries, frozen 1 cup, unthawed (147g)	81	0	3	19	0	0	1	7.3
Loquats, raw 1 large (20g)	9	0	0	2	0	0	0	0.4
Mammy-apple (mamey), raw 1 fruit, without refuse (846g)	431	0	0	102	0	0	127	25.4

Food Serving size	Cal.	Fat cal.	Prot.	Carb.	Fat	Chol.	Sod.	Fiber
Mangos, raw 1 cup, sliced (165g)	107	0	2	28	0	0	3	3.3
Melons, cantaloupe, raw 1 cup, cubes (160g)	56	0	2	13	0	0	14	1.6
Melons, casaba, raw 1 cup, cubes (170g)	44	0	2	10	0	0	20	1.7
Melons, honeydew, raw 1 cup, diced (approx 20 pieces per cup)	60	0	0	15	0	0	17	1.7
Mulberries, raw 10 fruits (15g)	6	0	0	2	0	0	2	0.3
Nectarines, raw 1 fruit ($2\frac{1}{2}''$ dia) (136g)	67	0	1	16	0	0	0	2.7
Olives, ripe, canned, jumbo-super colossal 1 jumbo (8g)	6	5	0	0	1	0	72	0.2
Olives, ripe, canned, small-extra large 1 large (4g)	5	4	0	0	0	0	35	0.1
Oranges, raw, all commercial varieties 1 cup, sections (180g)	85	0	2	22	0	0	0	3.6
Oranges, raw, California, navels 1 fruit ($2\frac{7}{8}''$ dia) (140g)	64	0	1	17	0	0	1	2.8
Oranges, raw, California, Valencias 1 fruit ($2\frac{5}{8}''$ dia) (121g)	59	0	1	15	0	0	0	2.4
Oranges, raw, Florida 1 fruit, ($2\frac{5}{8}''$ dia) (141g)	65	0	1	17	0	0	0	2.8
Papaya nectar, canned 1 fl oz (31g)	18	0	0	5	0	0	2	0.3
Papayas, raw 1 cup, cubes (140g)	55	0	1	14	0	0	4	2.8

Food Serving size	Cal.	Fat cal.	Prot.	Carb.	Fat	Chol.	Sod.	Fiber
Passion-fruit, (granadilla), purple, raw 1 fruit, without refuse (18g)	17	2	0	4	0	0	5	1.8
Peach nectar, canned, without added ascorbic acid 1 fl oz (31g)	17	0	0	4	0	0	2	0.3
Peaches, canned, extra heavy syrup pack, solids and liquids 1 cup halves or slices (262g)	252	0	0	68	0	0	21	2.6
Peaches, canned, extra light syrup, solids and liquids 1 cup halves or slices (247g)	104	0	0	27	0	0	12	2.5
Peaches, canned, heavy syrup pack, solids and liquids 1 half with liquid (98g)	73	0	0	20	0	0	6	1.0
Peaches, canned, juice pack, solids and liquids 1 cup halves or slices (248g)	109	0	2	30	0	0	10	2.5
Peaches, canned, light syrup pack, solids and liquids 1 half with liquid (98g)	53	0	0	15	0	0	5	1.0
Peaches, canned, water pack, solids and liquids 1 half with liquid (98g)	24	0	0	6	0	0	3	1.0
Peaches, raw 1 large ($2\frac{3}{4}''$ dia)	68	0	2	17	0	0	0	3.1
Pear nectar, canned, without added ascorbic acid 1 fl oz (31g)	19	0	0	5	0	0	1	0.3
Pears, Asian, raw 1 fruit, $2\frac{1}{4}''$ high x $2\frac{1}{2}''$ dia (122g)	51	0	0	13	0	0	0	4.9
Pears, canned, extra heavy syrup pack, solids and liquids 1 half, $1\frac{3}{4}$ tablespoon liquid (79g)	77	0	0	20	0	0	4	1.6
Pears, canned, extra light syrup pack, solids and liquids 1 half with liquid (76g)	36	0	0	9	0	0	2	1.5
Pears, canned, heavy syrup pack, solids and liquids 1 half with liquid (76g)	56	0	0	14	0	0	4	1.5
Pears, canned, juice pack, solids and liquids 1 half with liquid (76g)	38	0	0	10	0	0	3	1.5

Food Serving size	Cal.	Fat cal.	Prot.	Carb.	Fat	Chol.	Sod.	Fiber
Pears, canned, light syrup pack, solids and liquids								
1 half with liquid (76g)	43	0	0	11	0	0	4	1.5
Pears, canned, water pack, solids and liquids								
1 half with liquid (76g)	22	0	0	6	0	0	2	1.5
Pears, raw								
1 cup, slices (165g)	97	0	0	25	0	0	0	3.3
Persimmons, Japanese, dried 1 fruit, without refuse								
(34g)	93	3	0	25	0	0	1	4.8
Persimmons, Japanese, raw 1 fruit ($2\frac{1}{2}''$ dia)								
(168g)	118	0	2	32	0	0	2	6.7
Persimmons, native, raw 1 fruit, without refuse								
(25g)	32	0	0	9	0	0	0	
Pineapple, canned, extra heavy syrup pack, solids and liquids 1 cup, crushed, sliced,								
or chunks (260g)	216	0	0	57	0	0	3	2.6
Pineapple, canned, heavy syrup pack, solids and liquids 1 slice or ring (3″ dia)								
with liquid (49g)	38	0	0	10	0	0	0	0.5
Pineapple, canned, juice pack, solids and liquids 1 slice or ring (3″ dia)								
with liquid (47g)	28	0	0	8	0	0	0	0.5
Pineapple, canned, light syrup pack, solids and liquids 1 slice or ring (3″ dia)								
with liquid (48g)	25	0	0	6	0	0	0	0.5
Pineapple, canned, water pack, solids and liquids 1 slice or ring (3″ dia)								
with liquid (47g)	15	0	0	4	0	0	0	0.5
Pineapple, frozen, chunks, sweetened								
1 cup, chunks (245g)	208	0	0	54	0	0	5	2.5
Pineapple, raw								
1 cup, diced (155g)	76	0	0	19	0	0	2	1.5
Plantains, cooked								
1 cup, slices (154g)	179	0	2	48	0	0	8	3.1

Food Serving size	Cal.	Fat cal.	Prot.	Carb.	Fat	Chol.	Sod.	Fiber
Plums, canned, purple, extra heavy syrup pack, solids and liquids								
1 cup, pitted (261g)	264	0	0	68	0	0	50	2.6
Plums, canned, purple, heavy syrup pack, solids and liquids								
1 plum with liquid								
(46g)	41	0	0	11	0	0	9	0.5
Plums, canned, purple, juice pack, solids and liquids								
1 plum with liquid								
(46g)	27	0	0	7	0	0	0	0.5
Plums, canned, purple, light syrup pack, solids and liquids								
1 plum with liquid								
(46g)	29	0	0	7	0	0	9	0.5
Plums, canned, purple, water pack, solids and liquids								
1 plum with liquid								
(46g)	19	0	0	5	0	0	0	0.5
Plums, raw								
1 fruit ($2\frac{1}{8}''$ dia) (66g)	36	6	1	9	1	0	0	1.3
Pomegranates, raw								
1 pomegranate								
($3\frac{3}{8}''$ dia) (154g)	105	0	2	26	0	0	5	1.5
Prickly pears, raw								
1 fruit, without refuse								
(103g)	42	9	1	10	1	0	5	4.1
Prunes, canned, heavy syrup pack, solids and liquids								
5 fruits, 2 tablespoons								
liquid (86g)	90	0	1	24	0	0	3	3.4
Prunes, dried, stewed, with added sugar								
1 cup, pitted (248g)	308	0	2	82	0	0	5	9.9
Prunes, dried, stewed, without added sugar								
1 cup, pitted (248g)	265	0	2	69	0	0	5	17.4
Raisins, golden seedless								
1 cup (not packed)								
(145g)	438	0	4	116	0	0	17	5.8
Raisins, seeded								
1 cup (not packed)								
(145g)	429	12	4	113	1	0	41	10.1

Food Serving size	Cal.	Fat cal.	Prot.	Carb.	Fat	Chol.	Sod.	Fiber
Raisins, seedless 1 cup (not packed) (145g)	435	0	4	115	0	0	17	5.8
Raspberries, canned, red, heavy syrup pack, solids and liquids 1 cup (256g)	233	0	3	59	0	0	8	7.7
Raspberries, frozen, red, sweetened 1 cup, unthawed (250g)	258	0	3	65	0	0	3	10.0
Raspberries, raw 1 cup (123g)	60	10	1	15	1	0	0	8.6
Rhubarb, frozen, cooked, with sugar 1 cup (240g)	278	0	0	74	0	0	2	4.8
Rhubarb, raw 1 stalk (51g)	11	0	1	3	0	0	2	1.0
Strawberries, canned, heavy syrup pack, solids and liquids 1 cup (254g)	234	0	3	61	0	0	10	5.1
Strawberries, frozen, sweetened, sliced 1 cup, thawed (255g)	245	0	3	66	0	0	8	5.1
Strawberries, frozen, sweetened, whole 1 cup, thawed (255g)	199	0	3	54	0	0	3	5.1
Strawberries, frozen, unsweetened 1 cup, unthawed (149g)	52	0	0	13	0	0	3	3.0
Strawberries, raw 1 cup, halves (152g)	46	0	2	11	0	0	2	3.0
Tamarinds, raw 1 fruit, (3" x 1") (2g)	5	0	0	1	0	0	1	0.1
Tangerines (mandarin oranges), canned, juice pack 1 cup (249g)	92	0	2	25	0	0	12	2.5
Tangerines (mandarin oranges), canned, light syrup pack 1 cup (252g)	154	0	0	40	0	0	15	2.5
Tangerines (mandarin oranges), raw 1 large ($2\frac{1}{2}$" dia) (98g)	43	0	1	11	0	0	1	2.0
Watermelon, raw 1 cup, diced (152g)	49	0	2	11	0	0	3	0.0

Food Serving size	Cal.	Fat cal.	Prot.	Carb.	Fat	Chol.	Sod.	Fiber

Fruit Juices

Apple juice, canned or bottled, unsweetened, without added ascorbic acid

1 fl oz (31g)	15	0	0	4	0	0	1	0.0

Apple juice, frozen concentrate, unsweetened, diluted with 3 volume water without added ascorbic acid

1 fl oz (30g)	14	0	0	4	0	0	2	0.0

Grape juice, canned or bottled, unsweetened, without added vitamin C

1 fl oz (32g)	20	0	0	5	0	0	1	0.0

Grape juice, frozen concentrate, sweetened, diluted with 3 volume water, without added vitamin C

1 fl oz (31g)	16	0	0	4	0	0	1	0.0

Grapefruit juice, canned, sweetened

1 fl oz (31g)	14	0	0	3	0	0	1	0.0

Grapefruit juice, canned, unsweetened

1 fl oz (31g)	12	0	0	3	0	0	0	0.0

Grapefruit juice, frozen concentrate, unsweetened, diluted with 3 volume water

1 fl oz (31g)	13	0	0	3	0	0	0	0.0

Grapefruit juice, white, raw

1 fl oz (31g)	12	0	0	3	0	0	0	0.0

Lemon juice, canned or bottled

1 tablespoon (15g)	3	0	0	1	0	0	3	0.0

Lemon juice, raw

1 fl oz (30g)	8	0	0	3	0	0	0	0.0

Lime juice, canned or bottled, unsweetened

1 fl oz (31g)	7	0	0	2	0	0	5	0.0

Lime juice, raw

1 fl oz (31g)	8	0	0	3	0	0	0	0.0

Orange juice, canned, unsweetened

1 fl oz (31g)	13	0	0	3	0	0	1	0.0

Food Serving size	Cal.	Fat cal.	Prot.	Carb.	Fat	Chol.	Sod.	Fiber
Orange juice, raw								
1 fl oz (31g)	14	0	0	3	0	0	0	0.0
Orange-grapefruit juice, canned, unsweetened								
1 fl oz (31g)	13	0	0	3	0	0	1	0.0
Passion-fruit juice, purple, raw								
1 fl oz (31g)	16	0	0	4	0	0	2	0.0
Passion-fruit juice, yellow, raw								
1 fl oz (31g)	19	0	0	4	0	0	2	0.0
Pineapple juice, canned, unsweetened, without added ascorbic acid								
1 fl oz (31g)	17	0	0	4	0	0	0	0.0
Pineapple juice, frozen concentrate, unsweetened, diluted with 3 volume water								
1 fl oz (31g)	16	0	0	4	0	0	0	0.0
Pineapple juice, frozen concentrate, unsweetened, undiluted								
1 can (6 fl oz) (216g)	387	0	2	95	0	0	6	2.2
Prune juice, canned								
1 fl oz (32g)	23	0	0	5	0	0	1	0.3
Tangerine juice, canned, sweetened								
1 fl oz (31g)	16	0	0	4	0	0	0	0.0
Tangerine juice, frozen concentrate, sweetened, diluted with 3 volume water								
1 fl oz (30g)	14	0	0	3	0	0	0	
Tangerine juice, frozen concentrate, sweetened, undiluted								
1 can (6 fl oz) (214g)	345	0	4	83	0	0	6	2.1
Tangerine juice, raw								
1 fl oz (31g)	13	0	0	3	0	0	0	0.0

Dairy and Egg Products

Food Serving size	Cal.	Fat cal.	Prot.	Carb.	Fat	Chol.	Sod.	Fiber

Butter

Butter, whipped, with salt 1 tablespoon (9g)	65	64	0	0	7	20	74	0.0
Butter, with salt 1 tablespoon (14g)	100	100	0	0	11	31	116	0.0
Butter, without salt 1 tablespoon (14g)	100	100	0	0	11	31	2	0.0

For **Margarine,** *see* **Fats and Oils,** *page 63.*

Cheeses

Cheese fondue $\frac{1}{2}$ cup (108g)	247		15	4	14	49	143	0.0
Cheese food, cold pack, American 1 oz (28g)	93	59	6	2	7	18	270	0.0
Cheese food, pasteurized process, American 1 oz (28g)	92	62	6	2	7	18	333	0.0
Cheese food, pasteurized process, Swiss 1 oz (28g)	90	59	6	1	7	23	435	0.0
Cheese sauce, prepared from recipe 2 tablespoons (30g)	59	40	3	2	5	11	148	0.0

Food Serving size	Cal.	Fat cal.	Prot.	Carb.	Fat	Chol.	Sod.	Fiber
Cheese spread, pasteurized process, American								
1 cup, diced (140g)	406	258	22	13	29	77	1883	0.0
Cheese substitute, mozzarella								
1 oz (28g)	69	30	3	7	3	0	192	0.0
Cheese, blue								
1 cubic inch (17g)	60	43	4	0	5	13	237	0.0
Cheese, brick								
1 cup, shredded (113g)	419	298	26	3	34	106	633	0.0
Cheese, brie								
1 cup, sliced (144g)	481	354	30	0	40	144	906	0.0
Cheese, camembert								
1 oz (28g)	84	59	6	0	7	20	236	0.0
Cheese, caraway								
1 oz (28g)	105	71	7	1	8	26	193	0.0
Cheese, cheddar								
1 cup, diced (132g)	532	383	33	1	44	139	818	0.0
Cheese, cheshire								
1 oz (28g)	108	76	6	1	9	29	196	0.0
Cheese, colby								
1 cup, shredded (113g)	445	318	27	3	36	107	683	0.0
Cheese, cottage, 1% fat								
4 oz (113g)	81	10	14	3	1	5	459	0.0
Cheese, cottage, 2% fat								
4 oz (113g)	102	20	16	5	2	9	459	0.0
Cheese, cottage, creamed, large or small curd								
4 oz (113g)	116	50	14	3	6	17	458	0.0
Cheese, cottage, creamed, with fruit								
4 oz (113g)	140	30	11	15	3	12	458	0.0
Cheese, cottage, uncreamed, dry, large or small curd								
4 oz (113g)	96	0	19	2	0	8	15	0.0
Cheese, cream, fat free								
100 grams	96	9	14	6	1	8	545	0.0
Cheese, cream								
1 tablespoon (14g)	49	43	1	0	5	15	41	0.0

Food Serving size	Cal.	Fat cal.	Prot.	Carb.	Fat	Chol.	Sod.	Fiber
Cheese, Edam 1 oz (28g)	100	69	7	0	8	25	270	0.0
Cheese, feta 1 oz (28g)	74	52	4	1	6	25	312	0.0
Cheese, fontina 1 cup, shredded (108g)	420	294	28	2	33	125	864	0.0
Cheese, gjetost 1 oz (28g)	130	74	3	12	8	26	168	0.0
Cheese, goat, hard type 1 oz (28g)	127	89	9	1	10	29	97	0.0
Cheese, goat, semisoft type 1 oz (28g)	102	74	6	1	8	22	144	0.0
Cheese, goat, soft type 1 oz (28g)	75	52	5	0	6	13	103	0.0
Cheese, Gouda 1 oz (28g)	100	66	7	1	8	32	229	0.0
Cheese, Gruyere 1 cup, shredded (108g)	446	304	32	0	35	119	363	0.0
Cheese, Limburger 1 oz (28g)	92	66	6	0	8	25	224	0.0
Cheese, low fat, cheddar or colby 1 cup, shredded (113g)	195	70	27	2	8	24	692	0.0
Cheese, low sodium, cheddar or colby 1 cup, shredded (113g)	450	328	27	2	37	113	24	0.0
Cheese, Mexican, queso anejo 1 oz (28g)	104	74	6	1	8	29	317	0.0
Cheese, Mexican, queso asadero 1 cup, shredded (113g)	402	278	26	3	32	119	740	0.0
Cheese, Mexican, queso chihuahua 1 cup, shredded (113g)	423	298	25	7	34	119	697	0.0
Cheese, Monterey Jack 1 cup, shredded (113g)	421	298	27	1	34	101	606	0.0
Cheese, mozzarella, part skim milk, low moisture 1 cup, shredded (113g)	316	169	31	3	19	61	597	0.0

Food Serving size	Cal.	Fat cal.	Prot.	Carb.	Fat	Chol.	Sod.	Fiber
Cheese, mozzarella, part skim milk								
1 oz (28g)	71	39	7	1	4	16	130	0.0
Cheese, mozzarella, whole milk, low moisture								
1 cubic inch (18g)	57	40	4	0	5	16	75	0.0
Cheese, mozzarella, whole milk								
1 oz (28g)	79	54	5	1	6	22	104	0.0
Cheese, Muenster								
1 cup, shredded (113g)	416	298	26	1	34	108	710	0.0
Cheese, Neufchatel								
1 oz (28g)	73	57	3	1	6	21	112	0.0
Cheese, Parmesan, grated								
1 tablespoon (5g)	23	13	2	0	2	4	93	0.0
Cheese, Parmesan, hard								
1 cubic inch (10g)	39	23	4	0	3	7	160	0.0
Cheese, Parmesan, shredded								
1 tablespoon (5g)	21	12	2	0	1	4	85	0.0
Cheese, pasteurized process, American								
1 cubic inch (18g)	68	49	4	0	6	17	117	0.0
Cheese, pasteurized process, pimento								
1 cup, diced (140g)	525	381	31	3	43	132	1999	0.0
Cheese, pasteurized process, Swiss								
1 cubic inch (18g)	60	40	5	0	5	15	123	0.0
Cheese, Port Salut								
1 cup, shredded (113g)	398	278	27	1	32	139	603	0.0
Cheese, provolone								
1 oz (28g)	98	66	7	1	8	19	245	0.0
Cheese, ricotta, part skim milk								
1 oz (28g)	39	20	3	1	2	9	35	0.0
Cheese, ricotta, whole milk								
$\frac{1}{2}$ cup (124g)	216	142	14	4	16	63	104	0.0
Cheese, Romano								
1 oz (28g)	108	66	9	1	8	29	336	0.0
Cheese, Roquefort								
1 oz (28g)	103	76	6	1	9	25	507	0.0

Food Serving size	Cal.	Fat cal.	Prot.	Carb.	Fat	Chol.	Sod.	Fiber
Cheese, Swiss 1 cup, diced (132g)	496	313	37	4	36	121	343	0.0
Cheese, Tilsit 1 oz (28g)	95	64	7	1	7	29	211	0.0

Milk Products

Food Serving size	Cal.	Fat cal.	Prot.	Carb.	Fat	Chol.	Sod.	Fiber
Cream substitute, liquid, with hydrogenated vegetable oil and soy protein 1 fl oz (30g)	41	26	0	3	3	0	24	0.0
Cream substitute, powdered 1 teaspoon (2g)	11	6	0	1	1	0	4	0.0
Cream, fluid, half and half 1 tablespoon (15g)	20	16	0	1	2	6	6	0.0
Cream, fluid, heavy whipping 1 cup whipped (120g)	414	390	2	4	44	164	46	0.0
Cream, fluid, light whipping 1 cup whipped (120g)	350	327	2	4	37	133	41	0.0
Cream, fluid, light, coffee or table 1 tablespoon (15g)	29	25	0	1	3	10	6	0.0
Cream, fluid, medium, 25% fat 1 tablespoon (15g)	37	33	0	0	4	13	6	0.0
Cream, sour half and half, cultured 1 tablespoon (15g)	20	16	0	1	2	6	6	0.0
Cream, sour, cultured 1 tablespoon (12g)	26	22	0	0	3	5	6	0.0
Cream, whipped, cream topping, pressurized 1 tablespoon (3g)	8	6	0	0	1	2	4	0.0
Dessert topping, powdered, 1.5 ounce prepared with $\frac{1}{2}$ cup milk 1 tablespoon (4g)	8	4	0	1	0	0	3	0.0
Dessert topping, powdered amount to make 1 tablespoon (1g)	6	4	0	1	0	0	1	0.0
Dessert topping, pressurized 1 tablespoon (4g)	11	8	0	1	1	0	2	0.0

Food Serving size	Cal.	Fat cal.	Prot.	Carb.	Fat	Chol.	Sod.	Fiber
Dessert topping, semi solid, frozen								
1 tablespoon (4g)	13	9	0	1	1	0	1	0.0
Eggnog								
1 fl oz (32g)	43	20	1	4	2	19	17	0.0
Milk shakes, thick chocolate								
1 fl oz (28g)	33	7	1	6	1	3	31	0.0
Milk shakes, thick vanilla								
1 fl oz (28g)	31	7	1	5	1	3	27	0.0
Milk substitutes, fluid with hydrogenated vegetable oils								
1 fl oz (30g)	18	8	1	2	1	0	23	0.0
Milk, buttermilk, fluid, cultured, from skim milk								
1 fl oz (31g)	12	3	1	2	0	1	33	0.0
Milk, canned, condensed, sweetened								
1 fl oz (38g)	122	30	3	21	3	13	48	0.0
Milk, canned, evaporated, skim								
1 fl oz (32g)	25	0	3	4	0	1	37	0.0
Milk, canned, evaporated, whole, with added vitamin A								
1 fl oz (32g)	43	23	2	3	3	9	34	0.0
Milk, canned, evaporated, whole, without added vitamin A								
1 fl oz (32g)	43	23	2	3	3	9	34	0.0
Milk, chocolate beverage, hot cocoa, homemade								
1 fl oz (31g)	24		1	4	1	2	16	0.3
Milk, chocolate drink, fluid, commercial, 1% fat								
1 cup (250g)	158	22	8	25	3	8	153	0.0
Milk, chocolate drink, fluid, commercial, 2% fat								
1 fl oz (31g)	22	5	1	3	1	2	19	0.0
Milk, chocolate drink, fluid, commercial, whole								
1 fl oz (31g)	26	8	1	3	1	4	19	0.3
Milk, dry, skim, nonfat solids, instant, with added vitamin A								
1 cup (68g)	243	6	24	35	1	12	373	0.0
Milk, dry, skim, nonfat solids, instant, without added vitamin A								
1 cup (68g)	243	6	24	35	1	12	373	0.0
Milk, dry, skim, nonfat solids, regular, with added vitamin A								
$\frac{1}{4}$ cup (30g)	109	3	11	16	0	6	161	0.0

Food Serving size	Cal.	Fat cal.	Prot.	Carb.	Fat	Chol.	Sod.	Fiber
Milk, dry, skim, nonfat solids, regular, without added vitamin A								
$\frac{1}{4}$ cup (30g)	109	3	11	16	0	6	161	0.0
Milk, dry, whole								
$\frac{1}{4}$ cup (32g)	159	76	8	12	9	31	119	0.0
Milk, goat, fluid								
1 fl oz (30g)	21	11	1	1	1	3	15	0.0
Milk, human, mature, fluid								
1 fl oz (31g)	22	11	0	2	1	4	5	0.0
Milk, low fat, fluid, 1% fat, protein fortified, with added vitamin A								
1 cup (246g)	118	22	10	15	2	10	143	0.0
Milk, low fat, fluid, 1% fat, with added nonfat milk solids and vitamin A								
1 cup (245g)	105	22	7	12	2	10	127	0.0
Milk, low fat, fluid, 1% fat, with added vitamin A								
1 fl oz (30g)	13	3	1	2	0	1	15	0.0
Milk, low fat, fluid, 2% fat, protein fortified, with added vitamin A								
1 cup (246g)	138	43	10	12	5	20	145	0.0
Milk, low fat, fluid, 2% fat, with added nonfat milk solids and vitamin A								
1 cup (245g)	125	43	7	12	5	20	127	0.0
Milk, low fat, fluid, 2% fat, with added nonfat milk solids, without added vitamin A								
1 cup (245g)	137	43	10	12	5	20	145	0.0
Milk, low fat, fluid, 2% fat, with added vitamin A								
1 fl oz (30g)	15	5	1	2	1	2	15	0.0
Milk, low sodium, whole, fluid								
1 fl oz (30g)	18	8	1	1	1	4	1	0.0
Milk, skim, fluid, protein fortified, with added vitamin A								
1 cup (246g)	101	0	10	15	0	5	145	0.0
Milk, skim, fluid, with added nonfat milk solids and vitamin A								
1 fl oz (31g)	11	0	1	2	0	1	16	0.0
Milk, skim, fluid, with added vitamin A								
1 fl oz (31g)	11	0	1	2	0	1	16	0.0
Milk, skim, fluid, without added vitamin A								
1 cup (245g)	86	0	7	12	0	5	127	0.0

Food Serving size	Cal.	Fat cal.	Prot.	Carb.	Fat	Chol.	Sod.	Fiber
Milk, whole, fluid, 3.3% fat								
1 tablespoon (15g)	9	4	0	1	0	2	7	0.0
Sour cream, imitation, cultured								
1 oz (28g)	58	49	1	2	6	0	29	0.0
Sour dressing, non-butterfat, cultured, filled cream-type								
1 tablespoon (12g)	21	18	0	1	2	1	6	0.0

Yogurt

Food Serving size	Cal.	Fat cal.	Prot.	Carb.	Fat	Chol.	Sod.	Fiber
Yogurt, coffee and vanilla, low fat, 11 grams protein per 8 ounce								
1 8-oz container (227g)	193	20	11	32	2	11	150	0.0
Yogurt, fruit, low fat, 11 grams protein per 8 ounce								
$\frac{1}{2}$ container, 4-oz net weight (113g)	119	10	6	21	1	7	73	0.0
Yogurt, fruit, low fat, 10 grams protein per 8 ounce								
1 6-oz container (170g)	173	15	7	32	2	7	99	0.0
Yogurt, fruit, low fat, 9 grams protein per 8 ounce								
1 4.4-oz container (125g)	124	11	5	24	1	5	66	0.0
Yogurt, plain, low fat, 12 grams protein per 8 ounce								
1 8-oz container (227g)	143	40	11	16	5	14	159	0.0
Yogurt, plain, skim milk, 13 grams protein per 8 ounce								
1 8-oz container (227g)	127	0	14	18	0	5	173	0.0
Yogurt, plain, whole milk, 8 grams protein per 8 ounce								
1 8-oz container (227g)	138	60	7	11	7	30	104	0.0

Eggs

Food Serving size	Cal.	Fat cal.	Prot.	Carb.	Fat	Chol.	Sod.	Fiber
Egg, duck, whole, fresh, raw								
1 egg (70g)	130	88	9	1	10	619	102	0.0
Egg, goose, whole, fresh, raw								
1 egg (144g)	266	169	20	1	19	1227	199	0.0
Egg, quail, whole, fresh, raw								
1 egg (9g)	14	9	1	0	1	76	13	0.0
Egg, turkey, whole, fresh, raw								
1 egg (79g)	135	86	11	1	9	737	119	0.0

Food Serving size	Cal.	Fat cal.	Prot.	Carb.	Fat	Chol.	Sod.	Fiber
Egg, white, raw, fresh 1 large egg white (33g)	17	0	4	0	0	0	54	0.0
Egg, whole, cooked, fried 1 large egg (46g)	92	62	6	0	7	211	162	0.0
Egg, whole, cooked, hard-boiled 1 tablespoon (8g)	12	8	1	0	1	34	10	0.0
Egg, whole, cooked, omelet 1 tablespoon (15g)	23	15	2	0	2	53	41	0.0
Egg, whole, cooked, poached 1 large egg (50g)	75	45	6	1	5	212	140	0.0
Egg, whole, cooked, scrambled 1 tablespoon (14g)	23	15	2	0	2	49	39	0.0
Egg, whole, raw, fresh 1 extra large (58g)	86	52	7	1	6	247	73	0.0
Egg, yolk, raw, fresh 1 large egg yolk (17g)	61	48	3	0	5	218	7	0.0
Egg substitute, frozen $\frac{1}{4}$ cup (60g)	96	58	7	2	7	1	119	0.0
Egg substitute, liquid 1 tablespoon (16g)	13	4	2	0	0	0	28	0.0
Egg substitute, powder 0.35 oz (10g)	44	12	6	2	1	57	80	0.0

Cereal Grains and Pasta

Food Serving size	Cal.	Fat cal.	Prot.	Carb.	Fat	Chol.	Sod.	Fiber
Grains								
Barley, pearled, cooked 1 cup (157g)	193	0	3	44	0	0	5	6.3
Buckwheat groats, roasted 1 cup (168g)	155	14	5	34	2	0	7	5.0
Bulgur, cooked 1 tablespoon (8g)	7	0	0	2	0	0	0	0.3
Couscous, cooked 1 cup, cooked (157g)	176	0	6	36	0	0	8	1.6
Hominy, canned, white 1 cup (165g)	119	14	2	23	2	0	347	3.3
Hominy, canned, yellow 1 cup (160g)	115	13	2	22	2	0	336	3.2
Millet, cooked 1 cup (174g)	207	15	7	42	2	0	3	1.7
Oat bran, cooked 1 cup (219g)	88	18	7	24	2	0	2	6.6
Rice, brown, medium-grain, cooked 1 cup (195g)	218	16	4	47	2	0	2	3.9
Rice, white, long-grain, regular, cooked 1 cup (158g)	205	0	5	44	0	0	2	0.0

Food Serving size	Cal.	Fat cal.	Prot.	Carb.	Fat	Chol.	Sod.	Fiber
Rice, white, medium-grain, cooked 1 cup (186g)	242	0	4	54	0	0	0	0.0
Rice, white, with pasta, cooked 1 cup (202g)	246	51	6	42	6	2	1147	4.0
Wheat bran, crude 1 cup (58g)	125	19	9	38	2	0	1	24.9
Wheat germ, crude 1 cup (115g)	414	96	26	60	12	0	14	14.9
Wild rice, cooked 1 cup (164g)	166	0	7	34	0	0	5	3.3

Pasta

Food Serving size	Cal.	Fat cal.	Prot.	Carb.	Fat	Chol.	Sod.	Fiber
Macaroni, cooked, enriched 1 cup spiral shaped (134g)	189	11	7	38	1	0	1	1.3
Macaroni, cooked, unenriched 1 cup elbow shaped (140g)	197	12	7	39	1	0	1	1.4
Macaroni, protein-fortified, cooked, enriched $\frac{1}{2}$ cup (58g)	95	0	5	18	0	0	3	1.2
Macaroni, vegetable, cooked, enriched 1 cup (134g)	172	0	7	36	0	0	8	5.4
Macaroni, whole-wheat, cooked 1 cup elbow shaped (140g)	174	12	7	38	1	0	4	4.2
Noodles, Chinese, chow mein 1.5 oz (43g)	227	112	3	25	13	0	189	1.7
Noodles, egg, cooked, enriched 1 cup (160g)	213	13	8	40	2	53	11	1.6
Noodles, egg, cooked, unenriched, with added salt 1 cup (160g)	213	13	8	40	2	53	264	
Noodles, egg, cooked, unenriched, without added salt 1 cup (160g)	213	13	8	40	2	53	11	1.6
Noodles, egg, spinach, cooked, enriched 1 cup (160g)	211	27	8	38	3	53	19	3.2

Food Serving size	Cal.	Fat cal.	Prot.	Carb.	Fat	Chol.	Sod.	Fiber
Noodles, Japanese, soba, cooked 1 cup (114g)	113	0	6	24	0	0	68	
Noodles, Japanese, somen, cooked 1 cup (176g)	231	0	7	49	0	0	283	
Pasta, corn, cooked 1 cup (140g)	176	12	4	39	1	0	0	7.0
Pasta, fresh-refrigerated, plain, cooked 2 oz (57g)	75	5	3	14	1	19	3	
Pasta, fresh-refrigerated, spinach, cooked 2 oz (57g)	74	5	3	14	1	19	3	
Pasta, homemade, made with egg, cooked 2 oz (57g)	74	10	3	14	1	23	47	
Pasta, homemade, made without egg, cooked 2 oz (57g)	71	5	2	14	1	0	42	
Rice noodles, cooked 1 cup (176g)	192	0	2	44	0	0	33	1.8
Spaghetti, cooked, enriched, with added salt 1 cup (140g)	197	12	7	39	1	0	140	2.8
Spaghetti, cooked, unenriched, without added salt 1 cup (140g)	197	12	7	39	1	0	1	2.8
Spaghetti, protein-fortified, cooked, enriched 1 cup (140g)	230	0	11	45	0	0	7	2.8
Spaghetti, spinach, cooked 1 cup (140g)	182	12	7	36	1	0	20	
Spaghetti, whole-wheat, cooked 1 cup (140g)	174	12	7	38	1	0	4	5.6

Breakfast Cereals

Food Serving size	Cal.	Fat cal.	Prot.	Carb.	Fat	Chol.	Sod.	Fiber

Cold Cereals

Cereals ready-to-eat, 100% BRAN (wheat bran, barley)

	Cal.	Fat cal.	Prot.	Carb.	Fat	Chol.	Sod.	Fiber
1 oz (28g)	75	12	3	20	1	0	194	8.4

Cereals ready-to-eat, 40% BRAN FLAKES, RALSTON PURINA (wheat bran)

1 oz (28g)	91	2	3	22	0	0	261	3.9

Cereals ready-to-eat, BRAN CHEX (wheat bran, corn)

1 oz (28g)	89	7	3	22	1	0	197	4.5

Cereals ready-to-eat, CORN CHEX (corn)

1 oz (28g)	110	0	2	25	0	0	306	0.6

Cereals ready-to-eat, CORN FLAKES, RALSTON PURINA (corn)

1 cup (25g)	98	0	2	22	0	0	239	0.5

Cereals ready-to-eat, crispy rice (rice)

1 cup (28g)	111	0	2	25	0	0	206	0.3

Cereals ready-to-eat, FROSTED RICE KRINKLES (rice)

1 oz (28g)	108	0	1	25	0	0	176	0.3

Cereals ready-to-eat, GENERAL MILLS, CHEERIOS

1 cup (30g)	110		3	23	2	0	284	2.7

Cereals ready-to-eat, GENERAL MILLS, CINNAMON TOAST CRUNCH

$\frac{3}{4}$ cup (30g)	124		2	24	3	0	210	1.5

Cereals ready-to-eat, GENERAL MILLS, COCOA PUFFS

1 cup (30g)	119		1	27	1	0	181	0.3

Cereals ready-to-eat, GENERAL MILLS, COUNTRY CORN FLAKES

1 cup (30g)	114		2	26	1	0	284	0.6

Food Serving size	Cal.	Fat cal.	Prot.	Carb.	Fat	Chol.	Sod.	Fiber
Cereals ready-to-eat, GENERAL MILLS, CRISPY WHEATIES 'N RAISINS								
1 cup (55g)	191		4	45	1	0	285	3.3
Cereals ready-to-eat, GENERAL MILLS, FIBER ONE								
$\frac{1}{2}$ cup (30g)	62		3	24	1	0	143	14.4
Cereals ready-to-eat, GENERAL MILLS, FROSTED CHEERIOS								
100 grams	382		7	85	3	0	640	5.0
Cereals ready-to-eat, GENERAL MILLS, GOLDEN GRAHAMS								
$\frac{3}{4}$ cup (30g)	116		2	26	1	0	275	0.9
Cereals ready-to-eat, GENERAL MILLS, HONEY FROSTED WHEATIES								
$\frac{3}{4}$ cup (30g)	110		2	26	0	0	211	1.5
Cereals ready-to-eat, GENERAL MILLS, HONEY NUT CHEERIOS								
1 cup (30g)	115		3	24	1	0	259	1.5
Cereals ready-to-eat, GENERAL MILLS, KIX								
$1\frac{1}{3}$ cup (30g)	114		2	26	1	0	263	0.9
Cereals ready-to-eat, GENERAL MILLS, LUCKY CHARMS								
1 cup (30g)	116		2	25	1	0	203	1.2
Cereals ready-to-eat, GENERAL MILLS, MULTIGRAIN CHEERIOS								
1 cup (30g)	112		3	25	1	0	254	1.8
Cereals ready-to-eat, GENERAL MILLS, NATURE VALLEY TOASTED OATS GRANOLA								
$\frac{3}{4}$ cup (55g)	248		6	36	10	0	89	3.3
Cereals ready-to-eat, GENERAL MILLS, TOTAL (CORN FLAKES)								
$1\frac{1}{3}$ cup (30g)	112		2	26	1	0	203	0.6
Cereals ready-to-eat, GENERAL MILLS, TOTAL (RAISIN BRAN)								
1 cup (55g)	178		4	43	1	0	240	4.9
Cereals ready-to-eat, GENERAL MILLS, TOTAL								
$\frac{3}{4}$ cup (30g)	105		3	24	1	0	199	2.7
Cereals ready-to-eat, GENERAL MILLS, TRIX								
1 cup (30g)	122		1	26	2	0	197	0.6
Cereals ready-to-eat, GENERAL MILLS, WHEATIES								
1 cup (30g)	110		3	24	1	0	222	2.1
Cereals ready-to-eat, granola, homemade (oats, wheat germ)								
1 oz (28g)	131	60	4	15	7	0	7	2.8

Food Serving size	Cal.	Fat cal.	Prot.	Carb.	Fat	Chol.	Sod.	Fiber
Cereals ready-to-eat, HEALTHY CHOICE, KELLOGG'S ALMOND CRUNCH, with raisins								
1 cup (55g)	198		4	47	1	0	284	4.4
Cereals ready-to-eat, HEALTHY CHOICE, KELLOGG'S MULTI-GRAIN FLAKES								
1 cup (30g)	104		2	25	0	0	174	2.7
Cereals ready-to-eat, HEALTHY CHOICE, KELLOGG'S TOASTED BROWN SUGAR SQUARES								
1¼ cup (55g)	189		6	45	1	0	2	4.9
Cereals ready-to-eat, HEARTLAND NATURAL CEREAL, PLAIN (oats, wheat germ)								
1 oz (28g)	122	36	3	19	4	0	71	1.7
Cereals ready-to-eat, KELLOGG'S FROSTED MINI-WHEATS, regular and bite size								
1 cup, regular (51g)	173		5	42	1	0	2	5.6
Cereals ready-to-eat, KELLOGG, KELLOGG'S ALL-BRAN								
½ cup (30g)	79		4	23	1	0	61	9.6
Cereals ready-to-eat, KELLOGG, KELLOGG'S ALL-BRAN WITH EXTRA FIBER								
½ cup (30g)	53		4	23	1	0	127	15.3
Cereals ready-to-eat, KELLOGG, KELLOGG'S APPLE JACKS								
1 cup (30g)	116		2	27	0	0	134	0.6
Cereals ready-to-eat, KELLOGG, KELLOGG'S BRAN BUDS								
⅓ cup (30g)	83		3	24	1	0	200	12.0
Cereals ready-to-eat, KELLOGG, KELLOGG'S COCOA KRISPIES								
¾ cup (31g)	120		2	27	1	0	210	0.3
Cereals ready-to-eat, KELLOGG, KELLOGG'S COMPLETE BRAN FLAKES								
¾ cup (29g)	95		3	23	1	0	226	4.6
Cereals ready-to-eat, KELLOGG, KELLOGG'S CORN FLAKES								
1 cup (28g)	102		2	24	0	0	298	0.8
Cereals ready-to-eat, KELLOGG, KELLOGG'S CORN POPS								
1 cup (31g)	118		1	29	0	0	123	0.3
Cereals ready-to-eat, KELLOGG, KELLOGG'S CRACKLIN' OAT BRAN								
¾ cup (55g)	225		4	40	7	0	195	6.6

Food Serving size	Cal.	Fat cal.	Prot.	Carb.	Fat	Chol.	Sod.	Fiber
Cereals ready-to-eat, KELLOGG, KELLOGG'S FROOT LOOPS								
1 cup (30g)	117		2	26	1	0	141	0.6
Cereals ready-to-eat, KELLOGG, KELLOGG'S FROSTED FLAKES								
$\frac{3}{4}$ cup (31g)	119	0	1	28	0	0	200	0.6
Cereals ready-to-eat, KELLOGG, KELLOGG'S LOW FAT GRANOLA **without raisins**								
$\frac{1}{2}$ cup (55g)	213		4	44	3	0	135	3.3
Cereals ready-to-eat, KELLOGG, KELLOGG'S MUESLIX (Apple & **Almond Crunch)**								
$\frac{3}{4}$ cup (55g)	211		6	41	5	0	270	4.4
Cereals ready-to-eat, KELLOGG, KELLOGG'S NUT & HONEY **CRUNCH**								
$1\frac{1}{4}$ cup (55g)	223		4	46	2	0	370	1.1
Cereals ready-to-eat, KELLOGG, KELLOGG'S NUTRI-GRAIN **(Wheat)**								
$\frac{3}{4}$ cup (30g)	101		3	24	1	0	221	3.9
Cereals ready-to-eat, KELLOGG, KELLOGG'S PRODUCT 19								
1 cup (30g)	110		2	25	0	0	282	1.2
Cereals ready-to-eat, KELLOGG, KELLOGG'S RAISIN BRAN								
1 cup (61g)	186		5	47	1	0	354	7.9
Cereals ready-to-eat, KELLOGG, KELLOGG'S RICE KRISPIES **TREATS Cereal**								
$\frac{3}{4}$ cup (30g)	120		1	26	2	0	190	0.3
Cereals ready-to-eat, KELLOGG, KELLOGG'S RICE KRISPIES								
$1\frac{1}{4}$ cup (33g)	124		2	28	0	0	354	0.3
Cereals ready-to-eat, KELLOGG, KELLOGG'S SMACKS								
$\frac{3}{4}$ cup (27g)	103		2	24	1	0	51	1.1
Cereals ready-to-eat, KELLOGG, KELLOGG'S SPECIAL K								
1 cup (31g)	115		6	22	0	0	250	0.9
Cereals ready-to-eat, POST, HONEYBRAN (wheat)								
1 oz (28g)	95	5	3	23	1	0	162	3.1
Cereals ready-to-eat, QUAKER, CAP'N CRUNCH								
$\frac{3}{4}$ cup (27g)	107		1	23	1	0	208	0.8

Food Serving size	Cal.	Fat cal.	Prot.	Carb.	Fat	Chol.	Sod.	Fiber
Cereals ready-to-eat, QUAKER, QUAKER 100% NATURAL CEREAL with oats, honey, and raisins								
$\frac{1}{2}$ cup (51g)	218		5	36	7	1	11	3.6
Cereals ready-to-eat, QUAKER, QUAKER CRUNCHY BRAN								
$\frac{3}{4}$ cup (27g)	90		2	23	1	0	253	4.9
Cereals ready-to-eat, QUAKER, QUAKER FROSTED FLAKES								
$\frac{3}{4}$ cup (31g)	117		2	28	0	0	281	0.9
Cereals ready-to-eat, QUAKER, QUAKER OAT BRAN CEREAL								
$1\frac{1}{4}$ cup (57g)	213		9	42	3	0	205	5.7
Cereals ready-to-eat, QUAKER, QUAKER OAT LIFE (plain)								
$\frac{3}{4}$ cup (32g)	121		3	25	1	0	174	1.9
Cereals ready-to-eat, QUAKER, QUAKER PUFFED RICE								
1 cup (14g)	54		1	12	0	0	1	0.1
Cereals ready-to-eat, QUAKER, QUAKER PUFFED WHEAT								
$1\frac{1}{4}$ cup (15g)	55		2	11	0	0	1	1.4
Cereals ready-to-eat, QUAKER, QUAKER TOASTED OATMEAL CEREAL, HONEY NUT								
1 cup (49g)	191		5	39	3	0	166	3.4
Cereals ready-to-eat, RAISIN BRAN, RALSTON PURINA (wheat)								
$1\frac{1}{3}$ oz box (38g)	121	0	3	32	0	0	330	4.9
Cereals ready-to-eat, RICE CHEX (rice)								
1 oz (28g)	111	0	1	25	0	0	234	0.6
Cereals ready-to-eat, rice, puffed, fortified (rice)								
1 cup (14g)	56	0	1	13	0	0	0	0.3
Cereals ready-to-eat, SUGAR FROSTED FLAKES, RALSTON PURINA (corn)								
1 oz (28g)	109	2	1	25	0	0	182	0.6
Cereals ready-to-eat, WHEAT CHEX (wheat)								
1 oz (28g)	103	5	3	23	1	0	188	2.5
Cereals ready-to-eat, wheat germ, toasted, plain (wheat germ)								
1 oz (28g)	107	26	8	14	3	0	1	3.6
Cereals ready-to-eat, wheat, puffed, fortified (rice)								
1 cup (12g)	44	1	2	10	0	0	0	0.5

Food Serving size	Cal.	Fat cal.	Prot.	Carb.	Fat	Chol.	Sod.	Fiber
Cereals ready-to-eat, wheat, shredded, large biscuit (wheat) 1 rectangular biscuit (24g)	86	4	3	19	0	0	0	2.4
Cereals ready-to-eat, wheat, shredded, small biscuit (wheat) 1 oz (28g)	100	5	3	22	1	0	3	2.8

Hot Cereals

Food Serving size	Cal.	Fat cal.	Prot.	Carb.	Fat	Chol.	Sod.	Fiber
Cereals, corn grits, white, regular, quick, enriched, cooked with water, with salt (corn) $\frac{3}{4}$ cup (182g)	109	0	2	24	0	0	406	0.0
Cereals, corn grits, white, regular, quick, enriched, cooked with water, without salt (corn) 1 tablespoon (15g)	9	0	0	2	0	0	0	0.0
Cereals, CREAM OF RICE, cooked with water, with salt (rice) $\frac{3}{4}$ cup (183g)	95	0	2	22	0	0	317	0.0
Cereals, CREAM OF RICE, cooked with water, without salt (rice) 1 tablespoon (15g)	8	0	0	2	0	0	0	0.0
Cereals, CREAM OF WHEAT, regular, cooked with water, with salt (wheat) $\frac{3}{4}$ cup (188g)	100	0	4	21	0	0	252	1.9
Cereals, CREAM OF WHEAT, regular, cooked with water, without salt (wheat) 1 tablespoon (16g)	8	0	0	2	0	0	0	0.2
Cereals, farina, enriched, cooked with water, with salt (wheat) $\frac{3}{4}$ cup (175g)	88	0	2	19	0	0	576	1.8
Cereals, farina, enriched, cooked with water, without salt (wheat) 1 tablespoon (15g)	8	0	0	2	0	0	0	0.2
Cereals, MALT-O-MEAL, plain and chocolate, cooked with water, with salt (wheat, barley) $\frac{3}{4}$ cup (180g)	92	0	4	20	0	0	243	0.0
Cereals, MAYPO, cooked with water, with salt (oats with other grains) $\frac{3}{4}$ cup (180g)	128	15	4	23	2	0	194	3.6
Cereals, oats, instant, fortified, plain, prepared with water (oats) 1 cup, cooked (234g)	138	20	5	23	2	0	377	4.7

Food Serving size	Cal.	Fat cal.	Prot.	Carb.	Fat	Chol.	Sod.	Fiber
Cereals, oats, instant, fortified, with bran and raisins, prepared with water (oats, wheat bran)								
1 packet, prepared (195g)	158	16	4	31	2	0	248	5.8
Cereals, oats, instant, fortified, with cinnamon and spice, prepared with water (oats)								
1 tablespoon (15g)	17	1	0	3	0	0	26	0.3
Cereals, QUAKER, oatmeal, instant, maple and brown sugar, prepared with water								
1 packet, prepared (155g)	153		5	31	2	0	234	3.1
Cereals, QUAKER, oatmeal, microwave, QUICK 'N HEARTY Apple Spice								
1 packet (45g)	166		4	35	2	0	306	3.2
Cereals, RALSTON, cooked with water, with salt (oats)								
¾ cup (190g)	101	0	4	21	0	0	357	3.8
Cereals, ROMAN MEAL WITH OATS, cooked with water, with salt (wheat with other grains)								
¾ cup (180g)	128	15	5	25	2	0	405	5.4
Cereals, ROMAN MEAL WITH OATS, cooked with water, without salt (wheat with other grains)								
¾ cup (180g)	128	15	5	25	2	0	7	5.4
Cereals, ROMAN MEAL, plain, cooked with water, with salt (wheat with other grains)								
¾ cup (181g)	110	0	5	25	0	0	148	5.4
Cereals, ROMAN MEAL, plain, cooked with water, without salt (wheat with other grains)								
¾ cup (181g)	110	0	5	25	0	0	2	5.4
Cereals, WHEATENA, cooked with water (wheat)								
¾ cup (182g)	102	0	4	22	0	0	4	5.5
Cereals, WHEATENA, cooked with water, with salt (wheat)								
¾ cup (182g)	102	0	4	22	0	0	433	5.5
Cereals, whole wheat hot natural cereal, cooked with water, with salt (wheat)								
¾ cup (182g)	113	0	4	25	0	0	424	3.6

Food Serving size	Cal.	Fat cal.	Prot.	Carb.	Fat	Chol.	Sod.	Fiber
Cereals, whole wheat hot natural cereal, cooked with water, without salt (wheat)								
$\frac{3}{4}$ cup (182g)	113	0	4	25	0	0	0	3.6

Fats and Oils

Food Serving size	Cal.	Fat cal.	Prot.	Carb.	Fat	Chol.	Sod.	Fiber

Margarines

Margarine, regular, hard, coconut, hydrogenated and regular, and safflower and palm (hydrogenated)

1 teaspoon (5g)	36	35	0	0	4	0	47	0.0

Margarine, regular, hard, corn, hydrogenated and regular

1 teaspoon (5g)	36	35	0	0	4	0	47	0.0

Margarine, regular, hard, corn, hydrogenated

1 teaspoon (5g)	36	35	0	0	4	0	47	0.0

Margarine, regular, hard, corn and soybean, hydrogenated and cottonseed, hydrogenated, with salt

1 teaspoon (5g)	36	35	0	0	4	0	47	0.0

Margarine, regular, hard, corn and soybean, hydrogenated and cottonseed, hydrogenated, without salt

1 teaspoon (5g)	36	35	0	0	4	0	0	0.0

Margarine, regular, hard, lard, hydrogenated

1 teaspoon (5g)	37	36	0	0	4	3	47	0.0

Margarine, regular, hard, safflower and soybean, hydrogenated and regular, and cottonseed, hydrogenated

1 teaspoon (5g)	36	35	0	0	4	0	47	0.0

Margarine, regular, hard, safflower and soybean, hydrogenated, and cottonseed, hydrogenated

1 teaspoon (5g)	36	35	0	0	4	0	47	0.0

Margarine, regular, hard, safflower and soybean, hydrogenated

1 teaspoon (5g)	36	35	0	0	4	0	47	0.0

Food Serving size	Cal.	Fat cal.	Prot.	Carb.	Fat	Chol.	Sod.	Fiber
Margarine, regular, hard, soybean, hydrogenated and regular								
1 teaspoon (5g)	36	35	0	0	4	0	47	0.0
Margarine, regular, hard, soybean, hydrogenated, and corn and cottonseed, hydrogenated								
1 teaspoon (5g)	36	35	0	0	4	0	47	0.0
Margarine, regular, hard, soybean, hydrogenated, and cottonseed, hydrogenated								
1 teaspoon (5g)	36	35	0	0	4	0	47	0.0
Margarine, regular, hard, soybean, hydrogenated and cottonseed								
1 teaspoon (5g)	36	35	0	0	4	0	47	0.0
Margarine, regular, hard, soybean, hydrogenated and palm, hydrogenated and regular								
1 teaspoon (5g)	36	35	0	0	4	0	47	0.0
Margarine, regular, hard, soybean, hydrogenated, and palm, hydrogenated								
1 teaspoon (5g)	36	35	0	0	4	0	47	0.0
Margarine, regular, hard, soybean, hydrogenated, cottonseed, hydrogenated, and soybean								
1 teaspoon (5g)	36	35	0	0	4	0	47	0.0
Margarine, regular, hard, soybean, hydrogenated								
1 teaspoon (5g)	36	35	0	0	4	0	47	0.0
Margarine, regular, hard, soybean, soybean, hydrogenated, and cottonseed, hydrogenated								
1 teaspoon (5g)	36	35	0	0	4	0	47	0.0
Margarine, regular, hard, sunflower and soybean, hydrogenated, and cottonseed, hydrogenated								
1 teaspoon (5g)	36	35	0	0	4	0	47	0.0
Margarine, regular, liquid, soybean, hydrogenated and regular, and cottonseed								
1 tablespoon (14g)	101	100	0	0	11	0	109	0.0
Margarine, regular, unspecified oils, with salt added								
1 teaspoon (5g)	36	35	0	0	4	0	47	0.0
Margarine, regular, unspecified oils, without added salt								
1 teaspoon (5g)	36	35	0	0	4	0	0	0.0
Margarine, soft, corn, hydrogenated and regular								
1 teaspoon (5g)	36	35	0	0	4	0	54	0.0

Food Serving size	Cal.	Fat cal.	Prot.	Carb.	Fat	Chol.	Sod.	Fiber
Margarine, soft, safflower, hydrogenated and regular								
1 teaspoon (5g)	36	35	0	0	4	0	54	0.0
Margarine, soft, safflower and cottonseed, hydrogenated, and peanut, hydrogenated								
1 teaspoon (5g)	36	35	0	0	4	0	54	0.0
Margarine, soft, soybean, hydrogenated and regular, with salt								
1 teaspoon (5g)	36	35	0	0	4	0	54	0.0
Margarine, soft, soybean, hydrogenated and regular, without salt								
1 teaspoon (5g)	36	35	0	0	4	0	1	0.0
Margarine, soft, soybean, hydrogenated, and cottonseed, hydrogenated, with salt								
1 teaspoon (5g)	36	35	0	0	4	0	54	0.0
Margarine, soft, soybean, hydrogenated, and cottonseed, hydrogenated, without salt								
1 teaspoon (5g)	36	35	0	0	4	0	1	0.0
Margarine, soft, soybean, hydrogenated, and cottonseed								
1 teaspoon (5g)	36	35	0	0	4	0	54	0.0
Margarine, soft, soybean, hydrogenated, and palm, hydrogenated and regular								
1 teaspoon (5g)	36	35	0	0	4	0	54	0.0
Margarine, soft, soybean, hydrogenated, and safflower								
1 teaspoon (5g)	36	35	0	0	4	0	54	0.0
Margarine, soft, soybean, hydrogenated, cottonseed, hydrogenated, and soybean								
1 teaspoon (5g)	36	35	0	0	4	0	54	0.0
Margarine, soft, soybean, soybean, hydrogenated, and cottonseed, hydrogenated								
1 teaspoon (5g)	36	35	0	0	4	0	54	0.0
Margarine, soft, sunflower and cottonseed, hydrogenated, and peanut, hydrogenated								
1 teaspoon (5g)	36	35	0	0	4	0	54	0.0
Margarine, soft, unspecified oils, with salt added								
1 cup (227g)	1625	1605	2	0	182	0	2449	0.0
Margarine, soft, unspecified oils, without added salt								
1 teaspoon (5g)	36	35	0	0	4	0	1	0.0

Food Serving size	Cal.	Fat cal.	Prot.	Carb.	Fat	Chol.	Sod.	Fiber
Margarine-butter blend, 60% corn oil margarine and 40% butter								
1 tablespoon (14g)	101	100	0	0	11	12	126	0.0
Margarine-like spread (approximately 40% fat), corn, hydrogenated and regular								
1 teaspoon (5g)	17	17	0	0	2	0	48	0.0
Margarine-like spread (approximately 40% fat), soybean, hydrogenated, and cottonseed, hydrogenated								
1 teaspoon (5g)	17	17	0	0	2	0	48	0.0
Margarine-like spread (approximately 40% fat), soybean, hydrogenated, and cottonseed								
1 teaspoon (5g)	17	17	0	0	2	0	48	0.0
Margarine-like spread (approximately 40% fat), soybean, hydrogenated, and palm, hydrogenated and regular								
1 teaspoon (5g)	17	17	0	0	2	0	48	0.0
Margarine-like spread (approximately 40% fat), soybean, hydrogenated								
1 teaspoon (5g)	17	17	0	0	2	0	48	0.0
Margarine-like spread (approximately 40% fat), unspecified oils								
1 teaspoon (5g)	17	17	0	0	2	0	48	0.0
Margarine-like spread (approximately 60% fat), stick, soybean, hydrogenated, and palm, hydrogenated								
1 teaspoon (5g)	27	27	0	0	3	0	50	0.0
Margarine-like spread (approximately 60% fat), tub, soybean, hydrogenated, and palm, hydrogenated and regular								
1 teaspoon (5g)	27	27	0	0	3	0	50	0.0
Margarine-like spread (approximately 60% fat), tub, soybean, hydrogenated, and cottonseed, hydrogenated								
1 teaspoon (5g)	27	27	0	0	3	0	50	0.0
Margarine-like spread (approximately 60% fat), tub, unspecified oils								
1 teaspoon (5g)	27	27	0	0	3	0	50	0.0

Oils

Food Serving size	Cal.	Fat cal.	Prot.	Carb.	Fat	Chol.	Sod.	Fiber
Oil, fish, cod liver								
1 tablespoon (14g)	126	126	0	0	14	80	0	0.0
Oil, fish, herring								
1 tablespoon (14g)	126	126	0	0	14	107	0	0.0

Food Serving size	Cal.	Fat cal.	Prot.	Carb.	Fat	Chol.	Sod.	Fiber
Oil, fish, menhaden								
1 tablespoon (14g)	126	126	0	0	14	73	0	0.0
Oil, fish, menhaden, fully hydrogenated								
1 tablespoon (12g)	108	108	0	0	12	60	0	0.0
Oil, fish, salmon								
1 tablespoon (14g)	126	126	0	0	14	68	0	0.0
Oil, fish, sardine								
1 tablespoon (14g)	126	126	0	0	14	99	0	0.0
Oil, olive, salad or cooking								
1 tablespoon (14g)	124	124	0	0	14	0	0	0.0
Oil, peanut, salad or cooking								
1 tablespoon (14g)	124	124	0	0	14	0	0	0.0
Oil, sesame, salad or cooking								
1 tablespoon (14g)	124	124	0	0	14	0	0	0.0
Oil, soybean, salad or cooking, hydrogenated, and cottonseed								
1 tablespoon (14g)	124	124	0	0	14	0	0	0.0
Oil, soybean, salad or cooking, hydrogenated								
1 tablespoon (14g)	124	124	0	0	14	0	0	0.0
Oil, soybean, salad or cooking								
1 tablespoon (14g)	124	124	0	0	14	0	0	0.0
Oil, vegetable, almond								
1 tablespoon (14g)	124	124	0	0	14	0	0	0.0
Oil, vegetable, apricot kernel								
1 tablespoon (14g)	124	124	0	0	14	0	0	0.0
Oil, vegetable, avocado								
1 tablespoon (14g)	124	124	0	0	14		0	0.0
Oil, vegetable, canola								
1 tablespoon (14g)	124	124	0	0	14	0	0	0.0
Oil, vegetable, cocoa butter								
1 tablespoon (14g)	124	124	0	0	14	0	0	0.0
Oil, vegetable, coconut								
1 tablespoon (14g)	121	121	0	0	14	0	0	0.0
Oil, vegetable, corn, salad or cooking								
1 tablespoon (14g)	124	124	0	0	14	0	0	0.0

Food Serving size	Cal.	Fat cal.	Prot.	Carb.	Fat	Chol.	Sod.	Fiber
Oil, vegetable, cottonseed, salad or cooking								
1 tablespoon (14g)	124	124	0	0	14	0	0	0.0
Oil, vegetable, hazelnut								
1 tablespoon (14g)	124	124	0	0	14	0	0	0.0
Oil, vegetable, mustard								
1 tablespoon (14g)	124	124	0	0	14		0	0.0
Oil, vegetable, nutmeg butter								
1 tablespoon (14g)	124	121	0	0	14	0	0	0.0
Oil, vegetable, palm kernel								
1 tablespoon (14g)	121	121	0	0	14	0	0	0.0
Oil, vegetable, palm								
1 tablespoon (14g)	124	124	0	0	14	0	0	0.0
Oil, vegetable, rice bran								
1 tablespoon (14g)	124	124	0	0	14	0	0	0.0
Oil, vegetable, safflower, salad or cooking, linoleic (over 70%)								
1 tablespoon (14g)	124	124	0	0	14	0	0	0.0
Oil, vegetable, safflower, salad or cooking, oleic (over 70%)								
1 tablespoon (14g)	124	124	0	0	14	0	0	0.0
Oil, vegetable, soybean lecithin								
1 tablespoon (14g)	107	107	0	0	14	0	0	0.0
Oil, vegetable, sunflower, linoleic (60% and over)								
1 tablespoon (14g)	124	124	0	0	14	0	0	0.0
Oil, vegetable, sunflower, linoleic, hydrogenated								
1 tablespoon (14g)	124	124	0	0	14	0	0	0.0
Oil, vegetable, sunflower, linoleic (less than 60%)								
1 tablespoon (14g)	124	124	0	0	14	0	0	0.0
Oil, vegetable, sunflower, oleic (70% and over)								
1 tablespoon (14g)	124	124	0	0	14	0	0	0.0
Oil, vegetable, walnut								
1 tablespoon (14g)	124	124	0	0	14	0	0	0.0
Oil, wheat germ								
1 tablespoon (14g)	124	124	0	0	14	0	0	0.0

Food Serving size	Cal.	Fat cal.	Prot.	Carb.	Fat	Chol.	Sod.	Fiber

Salad Dressings

Salad dressing, blue and Roquefort cheese, commercial, regular, without salt

| 1 tablespoon (15g) | 76 | 69 | 1 | 1 | 8 | 3 | 5 | 0.0 |

Salad dressing, blue or Roquefort cheese, commercial, regular, with salt

| 1 tablespoon (15g) | 76 | 69 | 1 | 1 | 8 | 3 | 164 | 0.0 |

Salad dressing, French, commercial, regular, with salt

| 1 tablespoon (16g) | 69 | 58 | 0 | 3 | 7 | 0 | 219 | 0.0 |

Salad dressing, French, commercial, regular, without salt

| 100 grams | 430 | 362 | 1 | 18 | 41 | 0 | 0 | 0.0 |

Salad dressing, French, cottonseed oil, home recipe

| 1 tablespoon (14g) | 88 | 87 | 0 | 0 | 10 | 0 | 92 | 0.0 |

Salad dressing, French, diet, low fat, 5 calories per teaspoon, with salt

| 1 tablespoon (16g) | 21 | 8 | 0 | 4 | 1 | 0 | 126 | 0.0 |

Salad dressing, French, diet, low fat, 5 calories per teaspoon, without salt

| 1 tablespoon (16g) | 21 | 8 | 0 | 4 | 1 | 0 | 5 | 0.0 |

Salad dressing, French, home recipe

| 1 tablespoon (14g) | 88 | 87 | 0 | 0 | 10 | 0 | 92 | 0.0 |

Salad dressing, home recipe, cooked, with hard margarine

| 1 tablespoon (16g) | 25 | 14 | 1 | 2 | 2 | 0 | 117 | 0.0 |

Salad dressing, home recipe, cooked, with soft margarine

| 1 tablespoon (16g) | 25 | 14 | 1 | 2 | 2 | 0 | 117 | 0.0 |

Salad dressing, home recipe, cooked

| 1 tablespoon (16g) | 25 | 14 | 1 | 2 | 2 | 9 | 117 | 0.0 |

Salad dressing, home recipe, vinegar and oil

| 1 tablespoon (16g) | 72 | 71 | 0 | 0 | 8 | 0 | 0 | 0.0 |

Salad dressing, Italian, commercial, diet, 2 calories per teaspoon, with salt

| 1 tablespoon (15g) | 16 | 13 | 0 | 1 | 2 | 1 | 118 | 0.0 |

Food Serving size	Cal.	Fat cal.	Prot.	Carb.	Fat	Chol.	Sod.	Fiber
Salad dressing, Italian, commercial, diet, 2 calories per teaspoon, without salt								
1 tablespoon (15g)	16	13	0	1	2	1	5	0.0
Salad dressing, Italian, commercial, regular, with salt								
1 tablespoon (15g)	70	64	0	2	7	0	118	0.0
Salad dressing, Italian, commercial, regular, without salt								
1 tablespoon (15g)	70	64	0	2	7	10	5	0.0
Salad dressing, mayonnaise type, regular, with salt								
1 tablespoon (15g)	59	44	0	4	5	4	107	0.0
Salad dressing, mayonnaise, imitation, milk cream								
1 tablespoon (15g)	15	7	0	2	1	6	76	0.0
Salad dressing, mayonnaise, imitation, soybean without cholesterol								
1 tablespoon (14g)	67	59	0	2	7	0	49	0.0
Salad dressing, mayonnaise, imitation, soybean								
1 tablespoon (15g)	35	25	0	2	3	4	75	0.0
Salad dressing, mayonnaise, soybean and safflower oil, with salt								
1 tablespoon (14g)	100	98	0	0	11	8	80	0.0
Salad dressing, mayonnaise, soybean oil, with salt								
1 tablespoon (14g)	100	98	0	0	11	8	80	0.0
Salad dressing, mayonnaise, soybean oil, without salt								
1 tablespoon (14g)	100	98	0	0	11	8	4	0.0
Salad dressing, Russian, low calorie, with salt								
1 tablespoon (16g)	23	6	0	4	1	1	139	0.0
Salad dressing, Russian, with salt								
1 tablespoon (15g)	74	68	0	2	8	3	130	0.0
Salad dressing, sesame seed								
1 tablespoon (15g)	66	60	0	1	7	0	150	0.2
Salad dressing, thousand island, commercial, regular, with salt								
1 tablespoon (16g)	60	51	0	2	6	4	112	0.0
Salad dressing, thousand island, diet, low calorie, 10 calories per teaspoon, with salt								
1 tablespoon (15g)	24	15	0	2	2	2	150	0.2

Food Serving size	Cal.	Fat cal.	Prot.	Carb.	Fat	Chol.	Sod.	Fiber

Miscellaneous Fats

Fat, beef tallow
| 1 tablespoon (13g) | 117 | 117 | 0 | 0 | 13 | 14 | 0 | 0.0 |

Lard
| 1 tablespoon (13g) | 117 | 117 | 0 | 0 | 13 | 12 | 0 | 0.0 |

Sandwich spread, with chopped pickle, regular, unspecified oils
| 1 tablespoon (15g) | 58 | 45 | 0 | 3 | 5 | 11 | 150 | 0.0 |

Shortening bread, soybean (hydrogenated) and cottonseed
| 1 tablespoon (13g) | 115 | 115 | 0 | 0 | 13 | 0 | 0 | 0.0 |

Shortening cake mix, soybean (hydrogenated) and cottonseed (hydrogenated)
| 1 tablespoon (13g) | 115 | 115 | 0 | 0 | 13 | 0 | 0 | 0.0 |

Shortening frying (heavy duty), beef tallow and cottonseed
| 1 tablespoon (13g) | 117 | 117 | 0 | 0 | 13 | 13 | 0 | 0.0 |

Shortening frying (heavy duty), palm (hydrogenated)
| 1 tablespoon (13g) | 115 | 115 | 0 | 0 | 13 | 0 | 0 | 0.0 |

Shortening frying (heavy duty), soybean (hydrogenated), linoleic (less than 1%)
| 1 tablespoon (13g) | 115 | 115 | 0 | 0 | 13 | 0 | 0 | 0.0 |

Shortening frying (regular), soybean (hydrogenated) and cottonseed (hydrogenated)
| 1 tablespoon (13g) | 115 | 115 | 0 | 0 | 13 | 0 | 0 | 0.0 |

Shortening household soybean (hydrogenated) and palm
| 1 tablespoon (13g) | 115 | 115 | 0 | 0 | 13 | 0 | 0 | 0.0 |

Shortening, household, lard and vegetable oil
| 1 tablespoon (13g) | 117 | 117 | 0 | 0 | 13 | 7 | 0 | 0.0 |

Shortening, household, soybean (hydrogenated)-cottonseed (hydrogenated)
| 1 tablespoon (13g) | 115 | 115 | 0 | 0 | 13 | 0 | 0 | 0.0 |

Shortening, multipurpose, soybean (hydrogenated) and palm (hydrogenated)
| 1 tablespoon (13g) | 115 | 115 | 0 | 0 | 13 | 0 | 0 | 0.0 |

Nut and Seed Products

Food Serving size	Cal.	Fat cal.	Prot.	Carb.	Fat	Chol.	Sod.	Fiber
Nuts								
Nuts, acorns, dried 1 oz (28g)	143	73	2	15	9	0	0	
Nuts, acorns, raw 1 oz (28g)	108	56	2	11	7	0	0	
Nuts, almond butter, honey and cinnamon, with salt added 1 tablespoon (16g)	96	70	3	4	8	0	27	0.6
Nuts, almond butter, honey and cinnamon, without salt added 1 tablespoon (16g)	96	70	3	4	8	0	2	
Nuts, almond butter, plain, with salt added 1 tablespoon (16g)	101	79	2	3	9	0	72	0.6
Nuts, almond butter, plain, without salt added 1 tablespoon (16g)	101	79	2	3	9	0	2	0.6
Nuts, almond paste 1 oz (28g)	128	66	3	13	8	0	3	1.4
Nuts, almonds, dried, blanched 1 tablespoon (9g)	53	40	2	2	5	0	1	0.6
Nuts, almonds, dried, unblanched 1 cup, ground (95g)	560	413	19	19	49	0	10	10.4
Nuts, almonds, dry roasted, unblanched, with salt added 1 oz (22 whole kernels) (28g)	164	122	4	7	15	0	218	3.9

Food
Serving size	Cal.	Fat cal.	Prot.	Carb.	Fat	Chol.	Sod.	Fiber
Nuts, almonds, dry roasted, unblanched, without salt added								
1 cup (138g)	810	601	22	33	72	0	15	19.3
Nuts, almonds, honey roasted, unblanched								
1 oz (28g)	166	117	5	8	14	0	36	3.9
Nuts, almonds, oil roasted, blanched, with salt added								
1 oz (24 whole kernels)								
(28g)	172	134	5	5	16	0	217	3.1
Nuts, almonds, oil roasted, blanched, without salt added								
1 oz (24 whole kernels)								
(28g)	172	134	5	5	16	0	3	3.1
Nuts, almonds, oil roasted, unblanched, with salt added								
1 oz (22 whole kernels)								
(28g)	173	136	6	4	16	0	218	3.1
Nuts, almonds, oil roasted, unblanched, without salt added								
1 oz (22 whole kernels)								
(28g)	173	136	6	4	16	0	3	3.1
Nuts, almonds, toasted, unblanched								
1 oz (28g)	165	120	6	6	14	0	3	3.1
Nuts, beechnuts, dried								
1 oz (28g)	161	117	2	10	14	0	11	
Nuts, Brazil nuts, dried, unblanched								
1 oz (6-8 kernels) (28g)	184	155	4	4	18	0	1	1.4
Nuts, butternuts, dried								
1 oz (28g)	171	134	7	3	16	0	0	1.4
Nuts, cashew butter, plain, with salt added								
1 tablespoon (16g)	94	66	3	4	8	0	98	0.3
Nuts, cashew butter, plain, without salt added								
1 tablespoon (16g)	94	66	3	4	8	0	2	0.3
Nuts, cashew nuts, dry roasted, with salt added								
1 oz (28g)	161	108	4	9	13	0	179	0.8
Nuts, cashew nuts, dry roasted, without salt added								
1 tablespoon (9g)	52	35	1	3	4	0	1	0.3
Nuts, cashew nuts, oil roasted, with salt added								
1 oz (18 kernels) (28g)	161	112	4	8	13	0	175	1.1
Nuts, cashew nuts, oil roasted, without salt added								
1 oz (18 kernels) (28g)	161	112	4	8	13	0	5	1.1

Food Serving size	Cal.	Fat cal.	Prot.	Carb.	Fat	Chol.	Sod.	Fiber
Nuts, chestnuts, Chinese, boiled and steamed								
1 oz (28g)	43	2	1	10	0	0	1	
Nuts, chestnuts, Chinese, dried								
1 oz (28g)	102	5	2	22	1	0	1	
Nuts, chestnuts, Chinese, raw								
1 oz (28g)	63	2	1	14	0	0	1	
Nuts, chestnuts, Chinese, roasted								
1 oz (28g)	67	2	1	15	0	0	1	
Nuts, chestnuts, European, boiled and steamed								
1 oz (28g)	37	2	1	8	0	0	8	
Nuts, chestnuts, European, dried, peeled								
1 oz (28g)	103	9	1	22	1	0	10	
Nuts, chestnuts, European, dried, unpeeled								
1 oz (28g)	105	9	2	22	1	0	10	3.4
Nuts, chestnuts, European, raw, peeled								
1 oz (28g)	55	2	1	12	0	0	1	
Nuts, chestnuts, European, raw, unpeeled								
1 oz (28g)	60	5	1	13	1	0	1	2.2
Nuts, chestnuts, European, roasted								
1 oz (3 kernels) (28g)	69	5	1	15	1	0	1	1.4
Nuts, chestnuts, Japanese, boiled and steamed								
1 oz (28g)	16	0	0	4	0	0	1	
Nuts, chestnuts, Japanese, dried								
1 oz (28g)	101	2	1	23	0	0	10	
Nuts, chestnuts, Japanese, raw								
1 oz (28g)	43	2	1	10	0	0	4	
Nuts, chestnuts, Japanese, roasted								
1 oz (28g)	56	2	1	13	0	0	5	
Nuts, coconut cream, canned (liquid expressed from grated meat)								
1 tablespoon (19g)	36	29	1	2	3	0	10	0.4
Nuts, coconut cream, raw (liquid expressed from grated meat)								
1 tablespoon (15g)	50	44	1	1	5	0	1	0.3
Nuts, coconut meat, dried, not sweetened								
1 oz (28g)	185	152	2	7	18	0	10	4.5

Food Serving size	Cal.	Fat cal.	Prot.	Carb.	Fat	Chol.	Sod.	Fiber
Nuts, coconut meat, dried, sweetened, flaked, canned								
1 cup (77g)	341	206	2	32	25	0	15	3.1
Nuts, coconut meat, dried, sweetened, flaked, packaged								
1 cup, flaked (74g)	351	198	2	36	24	0	189	3.0
Nuts, coconut meat, dried, sweetened, shredded								
1 cup, shredded (93g)	466	272	3	45	33	0	244	3.7
Nuts, coconut meat, dried, toasted								
1 oz (28g)	166	110	1	12	13	0	10	
Nuts, coconut meat, raw								
1 cup, shredded (80g)	283	221	2	12	26	0	16	7.2
Nuts, coconut milk, canned (liquid expressed from grated meat and water)								
1 tablespoon (15g)	30	26	0	0	3	0	2	
Nuts, coconut milk, raw (liquid expressed from grated meat and water)								
1 tablespoon (15g)	35	30	0	1	4	0	2	0.3
Nuts, coconut water (liquid from coconuts)								
1 tablespoon (15g)	3	0	0	1	0	0	16	0.2
Nuts, filberts or hazelnuts, dried, blanched								
1 oz (28g)	188	157	4	4	19	0	1	1.7
Nuts, filberts or hazelnuts, dried, unblanched								
1 cup, ground (75g)	474	395	10	11	47	0	2	4.5
Nuts, filberts or hazelnuts, dry roasted, unblanched, with salt added								
1 oz (28g)	185	155	3	5	18	0	218	
Nuts, filberts or hazelnuts, dry roasted, unblanched, without salt added								
1 oz (28g)	185	155	3	5	18	0	1	2.0
Nuts, filberts or hazelnuts, oil roasted, unblanched, with salt added								
1 oz (28g)	185	150	4	5	18	0	220	1.7
Nuts, filberts or hazelnuts, oil roasted, unblanched, without salt added								
1 oz (28g)	185	150	4	5	18	0	1	1.7
Nuts, ginkgo nuts, canned								
1 cup (155g)	172	26	3	34	3	0	476	13.9

Food Serving size	Cal.	Fat cal.	Prot.	Carb.	Fat	Chol.	Sod.	Fiber
Nuts, ginkgo nuts, dried 1 oz (28g)	97	5	3	20	1	0	4	
Nuts, ginkgo nuts, raw 1 oz (28g)	51	5	1	11	1	0	2	
Nuts, hickory nuts, dried 1 oz (28g)	184	150	4	5	18	0	0	1.7
Nuts, macadamia nuts, dried 1 oz (11 whole kernels) (28g)	197	173	2	4	21	0	1	2.5
Nuts, macadamia nuts, oil roasted, with salt added 1 oz (10–12 kernels) (28g)	201	180	2	4	22	0	73	2.5
Nuts, macadamia nuts, oil roasted, without salt added 1 cup (28g)	201	180	2	4	22	0	2	2.5
Nuts, mixed nuts, dry roasted, with peanuts, with salt added 1 oz (28g)	166	120	5	7	14	0	187	2.5
Nuts, mixed nuts, dry roasted, with peanuts, without salt added 1 oz (28g)	166	120	5	7	14	0	3	2.5
Nuts, mixed nuts, oil roasted, with peanuts, with salt added 1 oz (28g)	173	131	5	6	16	0	183	2.5
Nuts, mixed nuts, oil roasted, with peanuts, without salt added 1 tablespoon (9g)	56	42	2	2	5	0	1	0.9
Nuts, mixed nuts, oil roasted, without peanuts, without salt added 1 oz (28g)	172	131	4	6	16	0	3	1.7
Nuts, mixed nuts, without peanuts, oil roasted, with salt added 1 oz (28g)	172	131	4	6	16	0	196	1.7
Nuts, pecans, dried 1 cup, halves (108g)	720	615	9	19	73	0	1	8.6
Nuts, pecans, dry roasted, with salt added 1 oz (28g)	185	152	2	6	18	0	218	2.5
Nuts, pecans, dry roasted, without salt added 1 oz (28g)	185	152	2	6	18	0	0	2.5
Nuts, pecans, oil roasted, with salt added 1 oz (15 halves) (28g)	192	166	2	4	20	0	212	2.0

Food Serving size	Cal.	Fat cal.	Prot.	Carb.	Fat	Chol.	Sod.	Fiber
Nuts, pecans, oil roasted, without salt added								
1 oz (15 halves) (28g)	192	166	2	4	20	0	0	2.0
Nuts, pilinuts-canarytree, dried								
1 oz (15 kernels) (28g)	201	187	3	1	22	0	1	
Nuts, pine nuts, pignolia, dried								
1 tablespoon (9g)	51	38	2	1	5	0	0	0.4
Nuts, pine nuts, pinyon, dried								
10 nuts (1g)	6	5	0	0	1	0	1	0.1
Nuts, pistachio nuts, dried								
1 oz (47 kernels) (28g)	162	112	6	7	13	0	2	3.1
Nuts, pistachio nuts, dry roasted, with salt added								
1 oz (28g)	170	124	4	8	15	0	218	3.1
Nuts, pistachio nuts, dry roasted, without salt added								
1 oz (28g)	170	124	4	8	15	0	2	3.1
Nuts, walnuts, black, dried								
1 tablespoon (8g)	49	38	2	1	5	0	0	0.4
Nuts, walnuts, English or Persian, dried								
1 cup, ground (80g)	514	415	11	14	50	0	8	4.0

Seeds

Food Serving size	Cal.	Fat cal.	Prot.	Carb.	Fat	Chol.	Sod.	Fiber
Seeds, breadfruit seeds, roasted								
1 oz (28g)	58	7	2	11	1	0	8	
Seeds, cottonseed flour, partially defatted								
1 tablespoon (5g)	18	3	2	2	0	0	2	0.2
Seeds, cottonseed kernels, roasted								
1 tablespoon (10g)	51	30	3	2	4	0	3	0.6
Seeds, cottonseed meal, partially defatted								
1 oz (28g)	103	12	14	11	1	0	10	
Seeds, lotus seeds, dried 1 oz (42 medium seeds) (28g)	93	5	4	18	1	0	1	
Seeds, lotus seeds, raw								
1 oz (28g)	25	2	1	5	0	0	0	

Food Serving size	Cal.	Fat cal.	Prot.	Carb.	Fat	Chol.	Sod.	Fiber
Seeds, pumpkin and squash seed kernels, dried 1 oz, hulled (142 seeds) (28g)	151	108	7	5	13	0	5	1.1
Seeds, pumpkin and squash seed kernels, roasted, with salt added 1 oz (28g)	146	98	9	4	12	0	161	1.1
Seeds, pumpkin and squash seed kernels, roasted, without salt 1 oz (28g)	146	98	9	4	12	0	5	1.1
Seeds, pumpkin and squash seeds, whole, roasted, with salt added 1 oz (85 seeds) (28g)	125	45	5	15	5	0	161	1.4
Seeds, pumpkin and squash seeds, whole, roasted, without salt 1 oz (85 seeds) (28g)	125	45	5	15	5	0	5	1.1
Seeds, safflower seed kernels, dried 1 oz (28g)	145	89	4	10	11	0	1	
Seeds, safflower seed meal, partially defatted 1 oz (28g)	96	5	10	14	1	0	1	
Seeds, sesame butter, paste 1 tablespoon (16g)	95	68	3	4	8	0	2	1.0
Seeds, sesame butter, tahini, from raw and stone ground kernels 1 tablespoon (15g)	86	60	3	4	7	0	11	1.4
Seeds, sesame butter, tahini, from roasted and toasted kernels (most common type) 1 tablespoon (15g)	89	68	3	3	8	0	17	1.4
Seeds, sesame seed kernels, dried 1 tablespoon (8g)	47	37	2	1	4	0	3	1.0
Seeds, sesame seed kernels, toasted, with salt added 1 oz (28g)	159	112	5	7	13	0	165	4.8
Seeds, sesame seed kernels, toasted, without salt added 1 oz (28g)	159	112	5	7	13	0	11	4.8
Seeds, sesame seeds, whole, dried 1 tablespoon (9g)	52	38	2	2	5	0	1	1.1
Seeds, sesame seeds, whole, roasted and toasted 1 oz (28g)	158	112	5	7	13	0	3	3.9
Seeds, sunflower seed butter, with salt added 1 tablespoon (16g)	93	64	3	4	8	0	83	

Food Serving size	Cal.	Fat cal.	Prot.	Carb.	Fat	Chol.	Sod.	Fiber
Seeds, sunflower seed butter, without salt								
1 tablespoon (16g)	93	64	3	4	8	0	0	
Seeds, sunflower seed kernels, dried								
1 cup, with hulls, edible								
yield (46g)	262	193	11	9	23	0	1	4.6
Seeds, sunflower seed kernels, dry roasted, with salt added								
1 oz (28g)	163	117	5	7	14	0	218	2.5
Seeds, sunflower seed kernels, dry roasted, without salt								
1 oz (28g)	163	117	5	7	14	0	1	3.1
Seeds, sunflower seed kernels, oil roasted, with salt added								
1 cup, hulled (135g)	830	644	28	20	77	0	814	9.4
Seeds, sunflower seed kernels, oil roasted, without salt								
1 oz (28g)	172	134	6	4	16	0	1	2.0
Seeds, sunflower seed kernels, toasted, with salt added								
1 oz (28g)	173	134	5	6	16	0	172	3.4
Seeds, sunflower seed kernels, toasted, without salt								
1 oz (28g)	173	134	5	6	16	0	1	3.4
Seeds, watermelon seed kernels, dried								
1 oz (28g)	156	110	8	4	13	0	28	

Beef Products

	Cal.	Fat cal.	Prot.	Carb.	Fat	Chol.	Sod.	Fiber

Beef cuts: Quarter-inch Trim

Beef, brisket, flat half, separable lean and fat, trimmed to $\frac{1}{4}''$ fat, all grades, braised

3 oz (85g)	309	215	21	0	24	81	48	0.0

Beef, brisket, flat half, separable lean only, trimmed to $\frac{1}{4}''$ fat, all grades, braised

3 oz (85g)	189	77	27	0	9	81	54	0.0

Beef, brisket, point half, separable lean and fat, trimmed to $\frac{1}{4}''$ fat, all grades, braised

3 oz (85g)	343	261	19	0	29	78	55	0.0

Beef, brisket, point half, separable lean only, trimmed to $\frac{1}{4}''$ fat, all grades, braised

3 oz (85g)	222	123	24	0	14	77	65	0.0

Beef, brisket, whole, separable lean and fat, trimmed to $\frac{1}{4}''$ fat, all grades, braised

3 oz (85g)	327	245	20	0	27	80	52	0.0

Beef, brisket, whole, separable lean only, trimmed to $\frac{1}{4}''$ fat, all grades, braised

3 oz (85g)	206	100	26	0	11	79	60	0.0

Beef, chuck, arm pot roast, separable lean and fat, trimmed to $\frac{1}{4}''$ fat, all grades, braised

3 oz (85g)	282	184	23	0	20	84	51	0.0

Beef, chuck, arm pot roast, separable lean and fat, trimmed to $\frac{1}{4}''$ fat, choice, braised

3 oz (85g)	296	199	23	0	22	84	50	0.0

Food Serving size	Cal.	Fat cal.	Prot.	Carb.	Fat	Chol.	Sod.	Fiber
Beef, chuck, arm pot roast, separable lean and fat, trimmed to $\frac{1}{4}''$ fat, select, braised								
3 oz (85g)	268	169	24	0	19	85	51	0.0
Beef, chuck, arm pot roast, separable lean only, trimmed to $\frac{1}{4}''$ fat, all grades, braised								
3 oz (85g)	184	61	28	0	7	86	56	0.0
Beef, chuck, arm pot roast, separable lean only, trimmed to $\frac{1}{4}''$ fat, choice, braised								
3 oz (85g)	191	69	28	0	8	86	56	0.0
Beef, chuck, arm pot roast, separable lean only, trimmed to $\frac{1}{4}''$ fat, select, braised								
3 oz (85g)	175	54	28	0	6	86	56	0.0
Beef, chuck, blade roast, separable lean and fat, trimmed to $\frac{1}{4}''$ fat, all grades, braised								
3 oz (85g)	293	199	23	0	22	88	54	0.0
Beef, chuck, blade roast, separable lean and fat, trimmed to $\frac{1}{4}''$ fat, choice, braised								
3 oz (85g)	309	215	22	0	24	88	54	0.0
Beef, chuck, blade roast, separable lean and fat, trimmed to $\frac{1}{4}''$ fat, select, braised								
3 oz (85g)	277	176	23	0	20	88	55	0.0
Beef, chuck, blade roast, separable lean only, trimmed to $\frac{1}{4}''$ fat, all grades, braised								
3 oz (85g)	213	100	26	0	11	90	60	0.0
Beef, chuck, blade roast, separable lean only, trimmed to $\frac{1}{4}''$ fat, choice, braised								
3 oz (85g)	224	107	26	0	12	90	60	0.0
Beef, chuck, blade roast, separable lean only, trimmed to $\frac{1}{4}''$ fat, select, braised								
3 oz (85g)	201	92	26	0	10	90	60	0.0
Beef, composite of trimmed retail cuts, separable lean and fat, trimmed to $\frac{1}{4}''$ fat, all grades, cooked								
3 oz (85g)	259	169	22	0	19	75	53	0.0
Beef, composite of trimmed retail cuts, separable lean and fat, trimmed to $\frac{1}{4}''$ fat, choice, cooked								
3 oz (85g)	274	184	21	0	20	75	52	0.0

Food Serving size	Cal.	Fat cal.	Prot.	Carb.	Fat	Chol.	Sod.	Fiber
Beef, composite of trimmed retail cuts, separable lean and fat, trimmed to $\frac{1}{4}''$ fat, prime, cooked								
3 oz (85g)	274	184	22	0	20	71	53	0.0
Beef, composite of trimmed retail cuts, separable lean and fat, trimmed to $\frac{1}{4}''$ fat, select, cooked								
3 oz (85g)	247	153	22	0	17	73	53	0.0
Beef, composite of trimmed retail cuts, separable lean only, trimmed to $\frac{1}{4}''$ fat, all grades, cooked								
3 oz (85g)	184	77	26	0	9	73	57	0.0
Beef, composite of trimmed retail cuts, separable lean only, trimmed to $\frac{1}{4}''$ fat, choice, cooked								
3 oz (85g)	189	84	26	0	9	73	57	0.0
Beef, composite of trimmed retail cuts, separable lean only, trimmed to $\frac{1}{4}''$ fat, prime, cooked								
3 oz (85g)	205	100	25	0	11	70	57	0.0
Beef, composite of trimmed retail cuts, separable lean only, trimmed to $\frac{1}{4}''$ fat, select, cooked								
3 oz (85g)	174	69	26	0	8	73	57	0.0
Beef, retail cuts, separable fat, cooked								
1 oz (28g)	190	177	3	0	20	27	11	0.0
Beef, rib, eye, small end (ribs 10–12), separable lean and fat, trimmed to $\frac{1}{4}''$ fat, choice, broiled								
3 oz (85g)	261	169	21	0	19	71	54	0.0
Beef, rib, eye, small end (ribs 10–12), separable lean only, trimmed to $\frac{1}{4}''$ fat, choice, broiled								
3 oz (85g)	191	92	24	0	10	68	59	0.0
Beef, rib, large end (ribs 6–9), separable lean and fat, trimmed to $\frac{1}{4}''$ fat, all grades, broiled								
3 oz (85g)	295	215	18	0	24	69	54	0.0
Beef, rib, large end (ribs 6–9), separable lean and fat, trimmed to $\frac{1}{4}''$ fat, all grades, roasted								
3 oz (85g)	310	230	20	0	26	72	54	0.0
Beef, rib, large end (ribs 6–9), separable lean and fat, trimmed to $\frac{1}{4}''$ fat, choice, broiled								
3 oz (85g)	312	238	18	0	26	69	54	0.0

Food Serving size	Cal.	Fat cal.	Prot.	Carb.	Fat	Chol.	Sod.	Fiber
Beef, rib, large end (ribs 6–9), separable lean and fat, trimmed to $\frac{1}{4}$″ fat, choice, roasted								
3 oz (85g)	326	245	19	0	27	72	54	0.0
Beef, rib, large end (ribs 6–9), separable lean and fat, trimmed to $\frac{1}{4}$″ fat, prime, broiled								
3 oz (85g)	351	276	17	0	31	73	52	0.0
Beef, rib, large end (ribs 6–9), separable lean and fat, trimmed to $\frac{1}{4}$″ fat, prime, roasted								
3 oz (85g)	342	261	19	0	29	72	54	0.0
Beef, rib, large end (ribs 6–9), separable lean and fat, trimmed to $\frac{1}{4}$″ fat, select, broiled								
3 oz (85g)	275	199	19	0	22	68	54	0.0
Beef, rib, large end (ribs 6–9), separable lean and fat, trimmed to $\frac{1}{4}$″ fat, select, roasted								
3 oz (85g)	289	207	20	0	23	72	55	0.0
Beef, rib, large end (ribs 6–9), separable lean only, trimmed to $\frac{1}{4}$″ fat, all grades, broiled								
3 oz (85g)	190	100	21	0	11	65	61	0.0
Beef, rib, large end (ribs 6–9), separable lean only, trimmed to $\frac{1}{4}$″ fat, all grades, roasted								
3 oz (85g)	201	100	24	0	11	69	62	0.0
Beef, rib, large end (ribs 6–9), separable lean only, trimmed to $\frac{1}{4}$″ fat, choice, broiled								
3 oz (85g)	204	115	21	0	13	65	61	0.0
Beef, rib, large end (ribs 6–9), separable lean only, trimmed to $\frac{1}{4}$″ fat, choice, roasted								
3 oz (85g)	213	115	24	0	13	69	62	0.0
Beef, rib, large end (ribs 6–9), separable lean only, trimmed to $\frac{1}{4}$″ fat, prime, broiled								
3 oz (85g)	250	161	21	0	18	70	60	0.0
Beef, rib, large end (ribs 6–9), separable lean only, trimmed to $\frac{1}{4}$″ fat, prime, roasted								
3 oz (85g)	241	138	24	0	15	69	62	0.0
Beef, rib, large end (ribs 6–9), separable lean only, trimmed to $\frac{1}{4}$″ fat, select, broiled								
3 oz (85g)	175	84	21	0	9	65	61	0.0

Food

Serving size	Cal.	Fat cal.	Prot.	Carb.	Fat	Chol.	Sod.	Fiber
Beef, rib, large end (ribs 6–9), separable lean only, trimmed to $\frac{1}{4}''$ fat, select, roasted								
3 oz (85g)	187	84	24	0	9	69	62	0.0
Beef, rib, small end (ribs 10–12), separable lean and fat, trimmed to $\frac{1}{4}''$ fat, all grades, broiled								
3 oz (85g)	286	199	20	0	22	71	53	0.0
Beef, rib, small end (ribs 10–12), separable lean and fat, trimmed to $\frac{1}{4}''$ fat, all grades, roasted								
3 oz (85g)	295	215	19	0	24	71	54	0.0
Beef, rib, small end (ribs 10–12), separable lean and fat, trimmed to $\frac{1}{4}''$ fat, choice, broiled								
3 oz (85g)	297	215	20	0	24	71	53	0.0
Beef, rib, small end (ribs 10–12), separable lean and fat, trimmed to $\frac{1}{4}''$ fat, choice, roasted								
3 oz (85g)	312	230	19	0	26	71	53	0.0
Beef, rib, small end (ribs 10–12), separable lean and fat, trimmed to $\frac{1}{4}''$ fat, prime, broiled								
3 oz (85g)	307	222	20	0	25	71	53	0.0
Beef, rib, small end (ribs 10–12), separable lean and fat, trimmed to $\frac{1}{4}''$ fat, prime, roasted								
3 oz (85g)	354	276	19	0	31	71	55	0.0
Beef, rib, small end (ribs 10–12), separable lean and fat, trimmed to $\frac{1}{4}''$ fat, select, broiled								
3 oz (85g)	273	184	20	0	20	71	53	0.0
Beef, rib, small end (ribs 10–12), separable lean and fat, trimmed to $\frac{1}{4}''$ fat, select, roasted								
3 oz (85g)	281	199	19	0	22	71	54	0.0
Beef, rib, small end (ribs 10–12), separable lean only, trimmed to $\frac{1}{4}''$ fat, all grades, broiled								
3 oz (85g)	188	84	24	0	9	68	59	0.0
Beef, rib, small end (ribs 10–12), separable lean only, trimmed to $\frac{1}{4}''$ fat, all grades, roasted								
3 oz (85g)	185	84	23	0	9	67	60	0.0
Beef, rib, small end (ribs 10–12), separable lean only, trimmed to $\frac{1}{4}''$ fat, choice, broiled								
3 oz (85g)	198	100	24	0	11	68	59	0.0

Food Serving size	Cal.	Fat cal.	Prot.	Carb.	Fat	Chol.	Sod.	Fiber
Beef, rib, small end (ribs 10–12), separable lean only, trimmed to $\frac{1}{4}$″ fat, choice, roasted								
3 oz (85g)	197	100	23	0	11	67	60	0.0
Beef, rib, small end (ribs 10–12), separable lean only, trimmed to $\frac{1}{4}$″ fat, prime, broiled								
3 oz (85g)	221	123	24	0	14	68	59	0.0
Beef, rib, small end (ribs 10–12), separable lean only, trimmed to $\frac{1}{4}$″ fat, prime, roasted								
3 oz (85g)	258	161	23	0	18	68	64	0.0
Beef, rib, small end (ribs 10–12), separable lean only, trimmed to $\frac{1}{4}$″ fat, select, broiled								
3 oz (85g)	176	77	24	0	9	68	59	0.0
Beef, rib, small end (ribs 10–12), separable lean only, trimmed to $\frac{1}{4}$″ fat, select, roasted								
3 oz (85g)	173	77	23	0	9	67	60	0.0
Beef, rib, whole (ribs 6–12), separable lean and fat, trimmed to $\frac{1}{4}$″ fat, all grades, broiled								
3 oz (85g)	291	207	19	0	23	70	54	0.0
Beef, rib, whole (ribs 6–12), separable lean and fat, trimmed to $\frac{1}{4}$″ fat, all grades, roasted								
3 oz (85g)	304	222	19	0	25	71	54	0.0
Beef, rib, whole (ribs 6–12), separable lean and fat, trimmed to $\frac{1}{4}$″ fat, choice, broiled								
3 oz (85g)	306	230	19	0	26	70	53	0.0
Beef, rib, whole (ribs 6–12), separable lean and fat, trimmed to $\frac{1}{4}$″ fat, choice, roasted								
3 oz (85g)	320	238	19	0	26	72	54	0.0
Beef, rib, whole (ribs 6–12), separable lean and fat, trimmed to $\frac{1}{4}$″ fat, prime, broiled								
3 oz (85g)	333	253	19	0	28	72	53	0.0
Beef, rib, whole (ribs 6–12), separable lean and fat, trimmed to $\frac{1}{4}$″ fat, prime, roasted								
3 oz (85g)	348	268	19	0	30	72	54	0.0
Beef, rib, whole (ribs 6–12), separable lean and fat, trimmed to $\frac{1}{4}$″ fat, select, broiled								
3 oz (85g)	275	192	19	0	21	70	54	0.0

Food Serving size	Cal.	Fat cal.	Prot.	Carb.	Fat	Chol.	Sod.	Fiber
Beef, rib, whole (ribs 6–12), separable lean and fat, trimmed to $\frac{1}{4}''$ fat, select, roasted								
3 oz (85g)	286	199	20	0	22	71	54	0.0
Beef, rib, whole (ribs 6–12), separable lean only, trimmed to $\frac{1}{4}''$ fat, all grades, broiled								
3 oz (85g)	190	92	22	0	10	65	60	0.0
Beef, rib, whole (ribs 6–12), separable lean only, trimmed to $\frac{1}{4}''$ fat, all grades, roasted								
3 oz (85g)	195	92	23	0	10	68	61	0.0
Beef, rib, whole (ribs 6–12), separable lean only, trimmed to $\frac{1}{4}''$ fat, choice, broiled								
3 oz (85g)	201	107	22	0	12	65	60	0.0
Beef, rib, whole (ribs 6–12), separable lean only, trimmed to $\frac{1}{4}''$ fat, choice, roasted								
3 oz (85g)	207	107	23	0	12	68	61	0.0
Beef, rib, whole (ribs 6–12), separable lean only, trimmed to $\frac{1}{4}''$ fat, prime, broiled								
3 oz (85g)	238	146	22	0	16	69	60	0.0
Beef, rib, whole (ribs 6–12), separable lean only, trimmed to $\frac{1}{4}''$ fat, prime, roasted								
3 oz (85g)	248	146	23	0	16	69	63	0.0
Beef, rib, whole (ribs 6–12), separable lean only, trimmed to $\frac{1}{4}''$ fat, select, broiled								
3 oz (85g)	175	77	22	0	9	65	60	0.0
Beef, rib, whole (ribs 6–12), separable lean only, trimmed to $\frac{1}{4}''$ fat, select, roasted								
3 oz (85g)	181	84	23	0	9	68	61	0.0
Beef, round, bottom round, separable lean and fat, trimmed to $\frac{1}{4}''$ fat, all grades, braised								
3 oz (85g)	234	130	25	0	14	82	43	0.0
Beef, round, bottom round, separable lean and fat, trimmed to $\frac{1}{4}''$ fat, all grades, roasted								
3 oz (85g)	211	115	23	0	13	68	54	0.0
Beef, round, bottom round, separable lean and fat, trimmed to $\frac{1}{4}''$ fat, choice, braised								
3 oz (85g)	241	138	25	0	15	82	43	0.0

Food Serving size	Cal.	Fat cal.	Prot.	Carb.	Fat	Chol.	Sod.	Fiber
Beef, round, bottom round, separable lean and fat, trimmed to $\frac{1}{4}''$ fat, choice, roasted								
3 oz (85g)	221	123	22	0	14	68	54	0.0
Beef, round, bottom round, separable lean and fat, trimmed to $\frac{1}{4}''$ fat, select, braised								
3 oz (85g)	220	115	25	0	13	82	43	0.0
Beef, round, bottom round, separable lean and fat, trimmed to $\frac{1}{4}''$ fat, select, roasted								
3 oz (85g)	199	100	23	0	11	68	54	0.0
Beef, round, bottom round, separable lean only, trimmed to $\frac{1}{4}''$ fat, all grades, braised								
3 oz (85g)	178	61	27	0	7	82	43	0.0
Beef, round, bottom round, separable lean only, trimmed to $\frac{1}{4}''$ fat, all grades, roasted								
3 oz (85g)	161	54	25	0	6	66	56	0.0
Beef, round, bottom round, separable lean only, trimmed to $\frac{1}{4}''$ fat, choice, braised								
3 oz (85g)	187	69	27	0	8	82	43	0.0
Beef, round, bottom round, separable lean only, trimmed to $\frac{1}{4}''$ fat, choice, roasted								
3 oz (85g)	168	61	25	0	7	66	56	0.0
Beef, round, bottom round, separable lean only, trimmed to $\frac{1}{4}''$ fat, select, braised								
3 oz (85g)	167	54	27	0	6	82	43	0.0
Beef, round, bottom round, separable lean only, trimmed to $\frac{1}{4}''$ fat, select, roasted								
3 oz (85g)	152	46	25	0	5	66	56	0.0
Beef, round, eye of round, separable lean and fat, trimmed to $\frac{1}{4}''$ fat, all grades, roasted								
3 oz (85g)	195	100	23	0	11	61	50	0.0
Beef, round, eye of round, separable lean and fat, trimmed to $\frac{1}{4}''$ fat, choice, roasted								
3 oz (85g)	205	107	23	0	12	61	50	0.0
Beef, round, eye of round, separable lean and fat, trimmed to $\frac{1}{4}''$ fat, select, roasted								
3 oz (85g)	184	84	23	0	9	61	51	0.0

Food Serving size	Cal.	Fat cal.	Prot.	Carb.	Fat	Chol.	Sod.	Fiber
Beef, round, eye of round, separable lean only, trimmed to $\frac{1}{4}''$ fat, all grades, roasted								
3 oz (85g)	143	38	25	0	4	59	53	0.0
Beef, round, eye of round, separable lean only, trimmed to $\frac{1}{4}''$ fat, choice, roasted								
3 oz (85g)	149	46	25	0	5	59	53	0.0
Beef, round, eye of round, separable lean only, trimmed to $\frac{1}{4}''$ fat, select, roasted								
3 oz (85g)	136	31	25	0	3	59	53	0.0
Beef, round, full cut, separable lean and fat, trimmed to $\frac{1}{4}''$ fat, choice, broiled								
3 oz (85g)	204	107	23	0	12	68	52	0.0
Beef, round, full cut, separable lean and fat, trimmed to $\frac{1}{4}''$ fat, select, broiled								
3 oz (85g)	190	92	23	0	10	47	53	0.0
Beef, round, full cut, separable lean only, trimmed to $\frac{1}{4}''$ fat, choice, broiled								
3 oz (85g)	162	54	25	0	6	66	54	0.0
Beef, round, full cut, separable lean only, trimmed to $\frac{1}{4}''$ fat, select, broiled								
3 oz (85g)	146	38	25	0	4	66	54	0.0
Beef, round, tip round, separable lean and fat, trimmed to $\frac{1}{4}''$ fat, all grades, roasted								
3 oz (85g)	199	100	23	0	11	70	54	0.0
Beef, round, tip round, separable lean and fat, trimmed to $\frac{1}{4}''$ fat, choice, roasted								
3 oz (85g)	210	115	23	0	13	71	53	0.0
Beef, round, tip round, separable lean and fat, trimmed to $\frac{1}{4}''$ fat, prime, roasted								
3 oz (85g)	233	138	22	0	15	71	53	0.0
Beef, round, tip round, separable lean and fat, trimmed to $\frac{1}{4}''$ fat, select, roasted								
3 oz (85g)	191	92	23	0	10	70	54	0.0
Beef, round, tip round, separable lean only, trimmed to $\frac{1}{4}''$ fat, all grades, roasted								
3 oz (85g)	157	54	25	0	6	69	55	0.0

Food Serving size	Cal.	Fat cal.	Prot.	Carb.	Fat	Chol.	Sod.	Fiber
Beef, round, tip round, separable lean only, trimmed to $\frac{1}{4}$″ fat, choice, roasted								
3 oz (85g)	160	54	25	0	6	69	55	0.0
Beef, round, tip round, separable lean only, trimmed to $\frac{1}{4}$″ fat, prime, roasted								
3 oz (85g)	181	77	25	0	9	69	55	0.0
Beef, round, tip round, separable lean only, trimmed to $\frac{1}{4}$″ fat, select, roasted								
3 oz (85g)	153	46	25	0	5	69	55	0.0
Beef, round, top round, separable lean and fat, trimmed to $\frac{1}{4}$″ fat, all grades, braised								
3 oz (85g)	211	84	29	0	9	77	38	0.0
Beef, round, top round, separable lean and fat, trimmed to $\frac{1}{4}$″ fat, all grades, broiled								
3 oz (85g)	184	77	26	0	9	72	51	0.0
Beef, round, top round, separable lean and fat, trimmed to $\frac{1}{4}$″ fat, choice, braised								
3 oz (85g)	221	100	29	0	11	77	38	0.0
Beef, round, top round, separable lean and fat, trimmed to $\frac{1}{4}$″ fat, choice, broiled								
3 oz (85g)	190	84	26	0	9	72	51	0.0
Beef, round, top round, separable lean and fat, trimmed to $\frac{1}{4}$″ fat, choice, pan-fried								
3 oz (85g)	235	115	27	0	13	82	58	0.0
Beef, round, top round, separable lean and fat, trimmed to $\frac{1}{4}$″ fat, prime, broiled								
3 oz (85g)	195	84	26	0	9	71	51	0.0
Beef, round, top round, separable lean and fat, trimmed to $\frac{1}{4}$″ fat, select, braised								
3 oz (85g)	199	77	29	0	9	77	38	0.0
Beef, round, top round, separable lean and fat, trimmed to $\frac{1}{4}$″ fat, select, broiled								
3 oz (85g)	175	69	26	0	8	72	51	0.0
Beef, round, top round, separable lean only, trimmed to $\frac{1}{4}$″ fat, all grades, braised								
3 oz (85g)	174	46	31	0	5	77	38	0.0

Food Serving size	Cal.	Fat cal.	Prot.	Carb.	Fat	Chol.	Sod.	Fiber
Beef, round, top round, separable lean only, trimmed to $\frac{1}{4}''$ fat, all grades, broiled								
3 oz (85g)	153	38	27	0	4	71	52	0.0
Beef, round, top round, separable lean only, trimmed to $\frac{1}{4}''$ fat, choice, braised								
3 oz (85g)	181	46	31	0	5	77	38	0.0
Beef, round, top round, separable lean only, trimmed to $\frac{1}{4}''$ fat, choice, broiled								
3 oz (85g)	161	46	27	0	5	71	52	0.0
Beef, round, top round, separable lean only, trimmed to $\frac{1}{4}''$ fat, choice, pan-fried								
3 oz (85g)	193	69	30	0	8	82	60	0.0
Beef, round, top round, separable lean only, trimmed to $\frac{1}{4}''$ fat, prime, broiled								
3 oz (85g)	183	69	27	0	8	71	52	0.0
Beef, round, top round, separable lean only, trimmed to $\frac{1}{4}''$ fat, select, braised								
3 oz (85g)	167	38	31	0	4	77	38	0.0
Beef, round, top round, separable lean only, trimmed to $\frac{1}{4}''$ fat, select, broiled								
3 oz (85g)	144	31	27	0	3	71	52	0.0
Beef, shank crosscuts, separable lean and fat, trimmed to $\frac{1}{4}''$ fat, choice, simmered								
3 oz (85g)	224	115	26	0	13	68	52	0.0
Beef, shank crosscuts, separable lean only, trimmed to $\frac{1}{4}''$ fat, choice, simmered								
3 oz (85g)	171	46	29	0	5	66	54	0.0
Beef, short loin, porterhouse steak, separable lean and fat, trimmed to $\frac{1}{4}''$ fat, all grades, broiled								
3 oz (85g)	273	192	20	0	21	62	54	0.0
Beef, short loin, porterhouse steak, separable lean and fat, trimmed to $\frac{1}{4}''$ fat, choice, broiled								
3 oz (85g)	278	199	19	0	22	64	53	0.0
Beef, short loin, porterhouse steak, separable lean and fat, trimmed to $\frac{1}{4}''$ fat, select, broiled								
3 oz (85g)	262	176	20	0	20	56	54	0.0

Food Serving size	Cal.	Fat cal.	Prot.	Carb.	Fat	Chol.	Sod.	Fiber
Beef, short loin, porterhouse steak, separable lean only, trimmed to $\frac{1}{4}''$ fat, all grades, broiled								
3 oz (85g)	180	84	22	0	9	56	59	0.0
Beef, short loin, porterhouse steak, separable lean only, trimmed to $\frac{1}{4}''$ fat, choice, broiled								
3 oz (85g)	183	92	22	0	10	59	59	0.0
Beef, short loin, porterhouse steak, separable lean only, trimmed to $\frac{1}{4}''$ fat, select, broiled								
3 oz (85g)	173	77	23	0	9	49	59	0.0
Beef, short loin, t-bone steak, separable lean and fat, trimmed to $\frac{1}{4}''$ fat, all grades, broiled								
3 oz (85g)	256	169	20	0	19	54	55	0.0
Beef, short loin, t-bone steak, separable lean and fat, trimmed to $\frac{1}{4}''$ fat, choice, broiled								
3 oz (85g)	263	176	20	0	20	57	54	0.0
Beef, short loin, t-bone steak, separable lean and fat, trimmed to $\frac{1}{4}''$ fat, select, broiled								
3 oz (85g)	238	146	21	0	16	49	56	0.0
Beef, short loin, t-bone steak, separable lean only, trimmed to $\frac{1}{4}''$ fat, all grades, broiled								
3 oz (85g)	173	77	23	0	9	48	60	0.0
Beef, short loin, t-bone steak, separable lean only, trimmed to $\frac{1}{4}''$ fat, choice, broiled								
3 oz (85g)	174	77	23	0	9	50	60	0.0
Beef, short loin, t-bone steak, separable lean only, trimmed to $\frac{1}{4}''$ fat, select, broiled								
3 oz (85g)	168	69	23	0	8	43	60	0.0
Beef, short loin, top loin, separable lean and fat, trimmed to $\frac{1}{4}''$ fat, all grades, broiled								
3 oz (85g)	244	153	22	0	17	67	54	0.0
Beef, short loin, top loin, separable lean and fat, trimmed to $\frac{1}{4}''$ fat, choice, broiled								
3 oz (85g)	253	161	21	0	18	67	54	0.0
Beef, short loin, top loin, separable lean and fat, trimmed to $\frac{1}{4}''$ fat, prime, broiled								
3 oz (85g)	275	184	21	0	20	67	54	0.0

Food Serving size	Cal.	Fat cal.	Prot.	Carb.	Fat	Chol.	Sod.	Fiber
Beef, short loin, top loin, separable lean and fat, trimmed to $\frac{1}{4}''$ fat, select, broiled								
3 oz (85g)	226	130	22	0	14	67	54	0.0
Beef, short loin, top loin, separable lean only, trimmed to $\frac{1}{4}''$ fat, all grades, broiled								
3 oz (85g)	176	69	25	0	8	65	58	0.0
Beef, short loin, top loin, separable lean only, trimmed to $\frac{1}{4}''$ fat, choice, broiled								
3 oz (85g)	182	77	25	0	9	65	58	0.0
Beef, short loin, top loin, separable lean only, trimmed to $\frac{1}{4}''$ fat, prime, broiled								
3 oz (85g)	208	107	25	0	12	65	58	0.0
Beef, short loin, top loin, separable lean only, trimmed to $\frac{1}{4}''$ fat, select, broiled								
3 oz (85g)	164	61	25	0	7	65	58	0.0
Beef, tenderloin, separable lean and fat, trimmed to $\frac{1}{4}''$ fat, all grades, broiled								
3 oz (85g)	247	153	21	0	17	73	50	0.0
Beef, tenderloin, separable lean and fat, trimmed to $\frac{1}{4}''$ fat, all grades, roasted								
3 oz (85g)	282	199	20	0	22	73	48	0.0
Beef, tenderloin, separable lean and fat, trimmed to $\frac{1}{4}''$ fat, choice, broiled								
3 oz (85g)	258	169	21	0	19	73	50	0.0
Beef, tenderloin, separable lean and fat, trimmed to $\frac{1}{4}''$ fat, choice, roasted								
3 oz (85g)	288	199	20	0	22	73	55	0.0
Beef, tenderloin, separable lean and fat, trimmed to $\frac{1}{4}''$ fat, prime, broiled								
3 oz (85g)	269	176	21	0	20	73	50	0.0
Beef, tenderloin, separable lean and fat, trimmed to $\frac{1}{4}''$ fat, prime, roasted								
3 oz (85g)	300	215	20	0	24	75	47	0.0
Beef, tenderloin, separable lean and fat, trimmed to $\frac{1}{4}''$ fat, select, broiled								
3 oz (85g)	230	138	22	0	15	73	51	0.0

Food Serving size	Cal.	Fat cal.	Prot.	Carb.	Fat	Chol.	Sod.	Fiber
Beef, tenderloin, separable lean and fat, trimmed to $\frac{1}{4}''$ fat, select, roasted								
3 oz (85g)	275	192	20	0	21	73	48	0.0
Beef, tenderloin, separable lean only, trimmed to $\frac{1}{4}''$ fat, all grades, broiled								
3 oz (85g)	179	77	24	0	9	71	54	0.0
Beef, tenderloin, separable lean only, trimmed to $\frac{1}{4}''$ fat, all grades, roasted								
3 oz (85g)	189	84	24	0	9	71	52	0.0
Beef, tenderloin, separable lean only, trimmed to $\frac{1}{4}''$ fat, choice, broiled								
3 oz (85g)	189	84	24	0	9	71	54	0.0
Beef, tenderloin, separable lean only, trimmed to $\frac{1}{4}''$ fat, choice, roasted								
3 oz (85g)	196	92	24	0	10	71	61	0.0
Beef, tenderloin, separable lean only, trimmed to $\frac{1}{4}''$ fat, prime, broiled								
3 oz (85g)	197	92	24	0	10	71	54	0.0
Beef, tenderloin, separable lean only, trimmed to $\frac{1}{4}''$ fat, prime, roasted								
3 oz (85g)	217	115	24	0	13	73	50	0.0
Beef, tenderloin, separable lean only, trimmed to $\frac{1}{4}''$ fat, select, broiled								
3 oz (85g)	169	69	24	0	8	71	54	0.0
Beef, tenderloin, separable lean only, trimmed to $\frac{1}{4}''$ fat, select, roasted								
3 oz (85g)	179	77	24	0	9	71	52	0.0
Beef, top sirloin, separable lean and fat, trimmed to $\frac{1}{4}''$ fat, all grades, broiled								
3 oz (85g)	219	115	24	0	13	77	54	0.0
Beef, top sirloin, separable lean and fat, trimmed to $\frac{1}{4}''$ fat, choice, broiled								
3 oz (85g)	229	130	24	0	14	77	53	0.0
Beef, top sirloin, separable lean and fat, trimmed to $\frac{1}{4}''$ fat, choice, pan-fried								
3 oz (85g)	277	176	24	0	20	83	60	0.0

Food Serving size	Cal.	Fat cal.	Prot.	Carb.	Fat	Chol.	Sod.	Fiber
Beef, top sirloin, separable lean and fat, trimmed to $\frac{1}{4}''$ fat, select, broiled								
3 oz (85g)	208	107	24	0	12	77	54	0.0
Beef, top sirloin, separable lean only, trimmed to $\frac{1}{4}''$ fat, all grades, broiled								
3 oz (85g)	166	54	26	0	6	76	56	0.0
Beef, top sirloin, separable lean only, trimmed to $\frac{1}{4}''$ fat, choice, broiled								
3 oz (85g)	172	61	26	0	7	76	56	0.0
Beef, top sirloin, separable lean only, trimmed to $\frac{1}{4}''$ fat, choice, pan-fried								
3 oz (85g)	202	84	27	0	9	84	65	0.0
Beef, top sirloin, separable lean only, trimmed to $\frac{1}{4}''$ fat, select, broiled								
3 oz (85g)	158	46	26	0	5	76	56	0.0

Beef cuts: Zero-inch Trim

Food Serving size	Cal.	Fat cal.	Prot.	Carb.	Fat	Chol.	Sod.	Fiber
Beef, brisket, flat half, separable lean and fat, trimmed to 0″ fat, all grades, braised								
3 oz (85g)	183	69	26	0	8	81	53	0.0
Beef, brisket, flat half, separable lean only, trimmed to 0″ fat, all grades, braised								
3 oz (85g)	162	46	27	0	5	81	54	0.0
Beef, brisket, point half, separable lean and fat, trimmed to 0″ fat, all grades, braised								
3 oz (85g)	304	215	20	0	24	78	58	0.0
Beef, brisket, point half, separable lean only, trimmed to 0″ fat, all grades, braised								
3 oz (85g)	207	107	24	0	12	77	65	0.0
Beef, brisket, whole, separable lean and fat, trimmed to 0″ fat, all grades, braised								
3 oz (85g)	247	153	23	0	17	79	55	0.0
Beef, brisket, whole, separable lean only, trimmed to 0″ fat, all grades, braised								
3 oz (85g)	185	77	26	0	9	79	60	0.0

Food Serving size	Cal.	Fat cal.	Prot.	Carb.	Fat	Chol.	Sod.	Fiber
Beef, chuck, arm pot roast, separable lean and fat, trimmed to 0″ fat, all grades, braised								
3 oz (85g)	238	130	26	0	14	85	53	0.0
Beef, chuck, arm pot roast, separable lean and fat, trimmed to 0″ fat, choice, braised								
3 oz (85g)	249	146	25	0	16	85	53	0.0
Beef, chuck, arm pot roast, separable lean and fat, trimmed to 0″ fat, select, braised								
3 oz (85g)	221	115	26	0	13	85	54	0.0
Beef, chuck, arm pot roast, separable lean only, trimmed to 0″ fat, all grades, braised								
3 oz (85g)	179	61	28	0	7	86	56	0.0
Beef, chuck, arm pot roast, separable lean only, trimmed to 0″ fat, choice, braised								
3 oz (85g)	186	69	28	0	8	86	56	0.0
Beef, chuck, arm pot roast, separable lean only, trimmed to 0″ fat, select, braised								
3 oz (85g)	168	46	28	0	5	86	56	0.0
Beef, chuck, blade roast, separable lean and fat, trimmed to 0″ fat, all grades, braised								
3 oz (85g)	284	184	23	0	20	88	55	0.0
Beef, chuck, blade roast, separable lean and fat, trimmed to 0″ fat, choice, braised								
3 oz (85g)	296	199	23	0	22	88	55	0.0
Beef, chuck, blade roast, separable lean and fat, trimmed to 0″ fat, select, braised								
3 oz (85g)	266	169	24	0	19	88	56	0.0
Beef, chuck, blade roast, separable lean only, trimmed to 0″ fat, all grades, braised								
3 oz (85g)	215	100	26	0	11	90	60	0.0
Beef, chuck, blade roast, separable lean only, trimmed to 0″ fat, choice, braised								
3 oz (85g)	225	115	26	0	13	90	60	0.0
Beef, chuck, blade roast, separable lean only, trimmed to 0″ fat, select, braised								
3 oz (85g)	202	92	26	0	10	90	60	0.0

Food Serving size	Cal.	Fat cal.	Prot.	Carb.	Fat	Chol.	Sod.	Fiber
Beef, composite of trimmed retail cuts, separable lean and fat, trimmed to 0″ fat, all grades, cooked								
3 oz (85g)	232	130	23	0	14	74	53	0.0
Beef, composite of trimmed retail cuts, separable lean and fat, trimmed to 0″ fat, choice, cooked								
3 oz (85g)	241	146	23	0	16	74	53	0.0
Beef, composite of trimmed retail cuts, separable lean and fat, trimmed to 0″ fat, select, cooked								
3 oz (85g)	222	123	23	0	14	73	54	0.0
Beef, composite of trimmed retail cuts, separable lean only, trimmed to 0″ fat, all grades, cooked								
3 oz (85g)	179	69	26	0	8	73	56	0.0
Beef, composite of trimmed retail cuts, separable lean only, trimmed to 0″ fat, choice, cooked								
3 oz (85g)	186	77	26	0	9	73	56	0.0
Beef, composite of trimmed retail cuts, separable lean only, trimmed to 0″ fat, select, cooked								
3 oz (85g)	171	61	26	0	7	73	56	0.0
Beef, flank, separable lean and fat, trimmed to 0″ fat, choice, braised								
3 oz (85g)	224	123	23	0	14	61	60	0.0
Beef, flank, separable lean and fat, trimmed to 0″ fat, choice, broiled								
3 oz (85g)	192	100	22	0	11	58	69	0.0
Beef, flank, separable lean only, trimmed to 0″ fat, choice, braised								
3 oz (85g)	201	100	24	0	11	60	61	0.0
Beef, flank, separable lean only, trimmed to 0″ fat, choice, broiled								
3 oz (85g)	176	77	23	0	9	57	71	0.0
Beef, rib, large end (ribs 6–9), separable lean and fat, trimmed to 0″ fat, all grades, roasted								
3 oz (85g)	300	215	20	0	24	72	55	0.0
Beef, rib, large end (ribs 6–9), separable lean and fat, trimmed to 0″ fat, choice, roasted								
3 oz (85g)	316	230	20	0	26	72	54	0.0
Beef, rib, large end (ribs 6–9), separable lean and fat, trimmed to 0″ fat, select, roasted								
3 oz (85g)	281	199	20	0	22	71	55	0.0

Food Serving size	Cal.	Fat cal.	Prot.	Carb.	Fat	Chol.	Sod.	Fiber
Beef, rib, large end (ribs 6–9), separable lean only, trimmed to 0″ fat, all grades, roasted								
3 oz (85g)	202	100	24	0	11	69	62	0.0
Beef, rib, large end (ribs 6–9), separable lean only, trimmed to 0″ fat, choice, roasted								
3 oz (85g)	215	115	24	0	13	69	62	0.0
Beef, rib, large end (ribs 6–9), separable lean only, trimmed to 0″ fat, select, roasted								
3 oz (85g)	187	84	24	0	9	69	62	0.0
Beef, rib, shortribs, separable lean and fat, choice, braised								
3 oz (85g)	400	322	19	0	36	80	43	0.0
Beef, rib, shortribs, separable lean only, choice, braised								
3 oz (85g)	251	138	26	0	15	79	49	0.0
Beef, rib, small end (ribs 10–12), separable lean and fat, trimmed to 0″ fat, all grades, broiled								
3 oz (85g)	252	161	21	0	18	71	54	0.0
Beef, rib, small end (ribs 10–12), separable lean and fat, trimmed to 0″ fat, choice, broiled								
3 oz (85g)	265	176	21	0	20	71	54	0.0
Beef, rib, small end (ribs 10–12), separable lean and fat, trimmed to 0″ fat, select, broiled								
3 oz (85g)	242	153	21	0	17	71	54	0.0
Beef, rib, small end (ribs 10–12), separable lean only, trimmed to 0″ fat, all grades, broiled								
3 oz (85g)	181	77	24	0	9	68	59	0.0
Beef, rib, small end (ribs 10–12), separable lean only, trimmed to 0″ fat, choice, broiled								
3 oz (85g)	191	92	24	0	10	68	59	0.0
Beef, rib, small end (ribs 10–12), separable lean only, trimmed to 0″ fat, select, broiled								
3 oz (85g)	168	69	24	0	8	68	59	0.0
Beef, round, bottom round, separable lean and fat, trimmed to 0″ fat, all grades, braised								
3 oz (85g)	181	69	26	0	8	82	43	0.0
Beef, round, bottom round, separable lean and fat, trimmed to 0″ fat, all grades, roasted								
3 oz (85g)	160	54	25	0	6	66	56	0.0

Food Serving size	Cal.	Fat cal.	Prot.	Carb.	Fat	Chol.	Sod.	Fiber
Beef, round, bottom round, separable lean and fat, trimmed to 0″ fat, choice, braised								
3 oz (85g)	193	84	26	0	9	82	43	0.0
Beef, round, bottom round, separable lean and fat, trimmed to 0″ fat, choice, roasted								
3 oz (85g)	173	69	24	0	8	66	55	0.0
Beef, round, bottom round, separable lean and fat, trimmed to 0″ fat, select, braised								
3 oz (85g)	171	61	26	0	7	82	43	0.0
Beef, round, bottom round, separable lean and fat, trimmed to 0″ fat, select, roasted								
3 oz (85g)	150	46	25	0	5	66	56	0.0
Beef, round, bottom round, separable lean only, trimmed to 0″ fat, all grades, braised								
3 oz (85g)	173	61	27	0	7	82	43	0.0
Beef, round, bottom round, separable lean only, trimmed to 0″ fat, all grades, roasted								
3 oz (85g)	156	54	25	0	6	66	56	0.0
Beef, round, bottom round, separable lean only, trimmed to 0″ fat, choice, braised								
3 oz (85g)	181	69	27	0	8	82	43	0.0
Beef, round, bottom round, separable lean only, trimmed to 0″ fat, choice, roasted								
3 oz (85g)	164	61	25	0	7	66	56	0.0
Beef, round, bottom round, separable lean only, trimmed to 0″ fat, select, braised								
3 oz (85g)	163	46	27	0	5	82	43	0.0
Beef, round, bottom round, separable lean only, trimmed to 0″ fat, select, roasted								
3 oz (85g)	145	38	25	0	4	66	56	0.0
Beef, round, eye of round, separable lean and fat, trimmed to 0″ fat, all grades, roasted								
3 oz (85g)	145	38	25	0	4	59	53	0.0
Beef, round, eye of round, separable lean and fat, trimmed to 0″ fat, choice, roasted								
3 oz (85g)	153	46	25	0	5	59	53	0.0

Food Serving size	Cal.	Fat cal.	Prot.	Carb.	Fat	Chol.	Sod.	Fiber
Beef, round, eye of round, separable lean and fat, trimmed to 0″ fat, select, roasted								
3 oz (85g)	137	31	25	0	3	59	53	0.0
Beef, round, eye of round, separable lean only, trimmed to 0″ fat, all grades, roasted								
3 oz (85g)	141	38	25	0	4	59	53	0.0
Beef, round, eye of round, separable lean only, trimmed to 0″ fat, choice, roasted								
3 oz (85g)	149	46	25	0	5	59	53	0.0
Beef, round, eye of round, separable lean only, trimmed to 0″ fat, select, roasted								
3 oz (85g)	132	31	25	0	3	59	53	0.0
Beef, round, tip round, separable lean and fat, trimmed to 0″ fat, all grades, roasted								
3 oz (85g)	162	61	24	0	7	69	54	0.0
Beef, round, tip round, separable lean and fat, trimmed to 0″ fat, choice, roasted								
3 oz (85g)	170	69	24	0	8	70	54	0.0
Beef, round, tip round, separable lean and fat, trimmed to 0″ fat, select, roasted								
3 oz (85g)	158	54	24	0	6	69	54	0.0
Beef, round, tip round, separable lean only, trimmed to 0″ fat, all grades, roasted								
3 oz (85g)	150	46	25	0	5	69	55	0.0
Beef, round, tip round, separable lean only, trimmed to 0″ fat, choice, roasted								
3 oz (85g)	153	46	25	0	5	69	55	0.0
Beef, round, tip round, separable lean only, trimmed to 0″ fat, select, roasted								
3 oz (85g)	145	38	25	0	4	69	55	0.0
Beef, round, top round, separable lean and fat, trimmed to 0″ fat, all grades, braised								
3 oz (85g)	178	46	31	0	5	77	38	0.0
Beef, round, top round, separable lean and fat, trimmed to 0″ fat, choice, braised								
3 oz (85g)	184	54	31	0	6	77	38	0.0

Food Serving size	Cal.	Fat cal.	Prot.	Carb.	Fat	Chol.	Sod.	Fiber
Beef, round, top round, separable lean and fat, trimmed to 0″ fat, select, braised								
3 oz (85g)	170	38	31	0	4	77	38	0.0
Beef, round, top round, separable lean only, trimmed to 0″ fat, all grades, braised								
3 oz (85g)	169	38	31	0	4	77	38	0.0
Beef, round, top round, separable lean only, trimmed to 0″ fat, choice, braised								
3 oz (85g)	176	46	31	0	5	77	38	0.0
Beef, round, top round, separable lean only, trimmed to 0″ fat, select, braised								
3 oz (85g)	162	31	31	0	3	77	38	0.0
Beef, short loin, porterhouse steak, separable lean and fat, trimmed to 0″ fat, all grades, broiled								
3 oz (85g)	237	153	20	0	17	57	55	0.0
Beef, short loin, porterhouse steak, separable lean and fat, trimmed to 0″ fat, choice, broiled								
3 oz (85g)	241	153	20	0	17	59	55	0.0
Beef, short loin, porterhouse steak, separable lean and fat, trimmed to 0″ fat, select, broiled								
3 oz (85g)	227	138	20	0	15	54	55	0.0
Beef, short loin, porterhouse steak, separable lean only, trimmed to 0″ fat, all grades, broiled								
3 oz (85g)	183	92	22	0	10	54	59	0.0
Beef, short loin, porterhouse steak, separable lean only, trimmed to 0″ fat, choice, broiled								
3 oz (85g)	190	100	22	0	11	55	59	0.0
Beef, short loin, porterhouse steak, separable lean only, trimmed to 0″ fat, select, broiled								
3 oz (85g)	165	69	23	0	8	49	59	0.0
Beef, short loin, t-bone steak, separable lean and fat, trimmed to 0″ fat, all grades, broiled								
3 oz (85g)	210	123	20	0	14	48	57	0.0
Beef, short loin, t-bone steak, separable lean and fat, trimmed to 0″ fat, choice, broiled								
3 oz (85g)	217	130	20	0	14	48	57	0.0

Food Serving size	Cal.	Fat cal.	Prot.	Carb.	Fat	Chol.	Sod.	Fiber
Beef, short loin, t-bone steak, separable lean and fat, trimmed to 0″ fat, select, broiled								
3 oz (85g)	194	107	20	0	12	49	58	0.0
Beef, short loin, t-bone steak, separable lean only, trimmed to 0″ fat, all grades, broiled								
3 oz (85g)	163	69	22	0	8	44	60	0.0
Beef, short loin, t-bone steak, separable lean only, trimmed to 0″ fat, choice, broiled								
3 oz (85g)	168	77	22	0	9	44	60	0.0
Beef, short loin, t-bone steak, separable lean only, trimmed to 0″ fat, select, broiled								
3 oz (85g)	150	54	22	0	6	46	60	0.0
Beef, short loin, top loin, separable lean and fat, trimmed to 0″ fat, all grades, broiled								
3 oz (85g)	180	77	24	0	9	65	57	0.0
Beef, short loin, top loin, separable lean and fat, trimmed to 0″ fat, choice, broiled								
3 oz (85g)	194	92	24	0	10	65	57	0.0
Beef, short loin, top loin, separable lean and fat, trimmed to 0″ fat, select, broiled								
3 oz (85g)	169	69	24	0	8	65	57	0.0
Beef, short loin, top loin, separable lean only, trimmed to 0″ fat, all grades, broiled								
3 oz (85g)	168	61	25	0	7	65	58	0.0
Beef, short loin, top loin, separable lean only, trimmed to 0″ fat, choice, broiled								
3 oz (85g)	178	77	25	0	9	65	58	0.0
Beef, short loin, top loin, separable lean only, trimmed to 0″ fat, select, broiled								
3 oz (85g)	156	54	25	0	6	65	58	0.0
Beef, tenderloin, separable lean and fat, trimmed to 0″ fat, all grades, broiled								
3 oz (85g)	200	100	23	0	11	72	53	0.0
Beef, tenderloin, separable lean and fat, trimmed to 0″ fat, choice, broiled								
3 oz (85g)	207	107	23	0	12	72	52	0.0

Food Serving size	Cal.	Fat cal.	Prot.	Carb.	Fat	Chol.	Sod.	Fiber
Beef, tenderloin, separable lean and fat, trimmed to 0" fat, select, broiled								
3 oz (85g)	195	92	23	0	10	72	53	0.0
Beef, tenderloin, separable lean only, trimmed to 0" fat, all grades, broiled								
3 oz (85g)	175	77	24	0	9	71	54	0.0
Beef, tenderloin, separable lean only, trimmed to 0" fat, choice, broiled								
3 oz (85g)	180	77	24	0	9	71	54	0.0
Beef, tenderloin, separable lean only, trimmed to 0" fat, select, broiled								
3 oz (85g)	170	69	24	0	8	71	54	0.0
Beef, top sirloin, separable lean and fat, trimmed to 0" fat, all grades, broiled								
3 oz (85g)	183	77	25	0	9	76	55	0.0
Beef, top sirloin, separable lean and fat, trimmed to 0" fat, choice, broiled								
3 oz (85g)	195	92	25	0	10	76	54	0.0
Beef, top sirloin, separable lean and fat, trimmed to 0" fat, select, broiled								
3 oz (85g)	166	61	26	0	7	76	55	0.0
Beef, top sirloin, separable lean only, trimmed to 0" fat, all grades, broiled								
3 oz (85g)	162	54	26	0	6	76	56	0.0
Beef, top sirloin, separable lean only, trimmed to 0" fat, choice, broiled								
3 oz (85g)	170	61	26	0	7	76	56	0.0
Beef, top sirloin, separable lean only, trimmed to 0" fat, select, broiled								
3 oz (85g)	153	46	26	0	5	76	56	0.0

Ground Beef

Food Serving size	Cal.	Fat cal.	Prot.	Carb.	Fat	Chol.	Sod.	Fiber
Beef, ground, extra lean, baked, medium								
3 oz (85g)	213	123	20	0	14	70	42	0.0
Beef, ground, extra lean, baked, well done								
3 oz (85g)	233	123	26	0	14	91	54	0.0

Food Serving size	Cal.	Fat cal.	Prot.	Carb.	Fat	Chol.	Sod.	Fiber
Beef, ground, extra lean, broiled, medium								
3 oz (85g)	218	123	21	0	14	71	60	0.0
Beef, ground, extra lean, broiled, well done								
3 oz (85g)	225	123	25	0	14	84	70	0.0
Beef, ground, extra lean, pan-fried, medium								
3 oz (85g)	217	123	21	0	14	69	60	0.0
Beef, ground, extra lean, pan-fried, well done								
3 oz (85g)	224	123	24	0	14	79	69	0.0
Beef, ground, lean, baked, medium								
3 oz (85g)	228	138	20	0	15	66	48	0.0
Beef, ground, lean, baked, well done								
3 oz (85g)	248	138	26	0	15	84	60	0.0
Beef, ground, lean, broiled, medium								
3 oz (85g)	231	138	21	0	15	74	65	0.0
Beef, ground, lean, broiled, well done								
3 oz (85g)	238	138	24	0	15	86	76	0.0
Beef, ground, lean, pan-fried, medium								
3 oz (85g)	234	146	20	0	16	71	65	0.0
Beef, ground, lean, pan-fried, well done								
3 oz (85g)	235	138	24	0	15	81	74	0.0
Beef, ground, patties, frozen, broiled, medium								
3 oz (85g)	240	153	20	0	17	80	65	0.0
Beef, ground, regular, baked, medium								
3 oz (85g)	244	161	20	0	18	74	51	0.0
Beef, ground, regular, baked, well done								
3 oz (85g)	269	161	25	0	18	92	64	0.0
Beef, ground, regular, broiled, medium								
3 oz (85g)	246	161	20	0	18	77	71	0.0
Beef, ground, regular, broiled, well done								
3 oz (85g)	248	146	23	0	16	86	79	0.0
Beef, ground, regular, pan-fried, medium								
3 oz (85g)	260	176	20	0	20	76	71	0.0
Beef, ground, regular, pan-fried, well done								
3 oz (85g)	243	146	23	0	16	83	79	0.0

Food Serving size	Cal.	Fat cal.	Prot.	Carb.	Fat	Chol.	Sod.	Fiber
Beef, ground, regular, (approximately 27% fat), raw								
1 oz (28g)	87	68	5	0	8	24	19	0.0

Variety Meats

Beef, variety meats and by-products, liver, braised								
3 oz (85g)	137	38	20	3	4	331	60	0.0
Beef, variety meats and by-products, liver, pan-fried								
3 oz (85g)	184	61	23	7	7	410	90	0.0
Beef, variety meats and by-products, tongue, simmered								
3 oz (85g)	241	161	19	0	18	91	51	0.0

Cured Beef

Beef, cured, breakfast strips, cooked								
3 slices (34g)	153	104	11	0	12	40	766	0.0
Beef, cured, corned beef, brisket, cooked								
3 oz (85g)	213	146	15	0	16	83	964	0.0

Fish and Shellfish Products

Food Serving size	Cal.	Fat cal.	Prot.	Carb.	Fat	Chol.	Sod.	Fiber

Fish

Anchovy, European, canned in oil, drained solids

1 anchovy (4g)	8	4	1	0	0	3	147	0.0

Bass, freshwater, mixed species, cooked, dry heat

1 fillet (62g)	91	28	15	0	3	54	56	0.0

Bass, striped, cooked, dry heat

3 oz (85g)	105	23	20	0	3	88	75	0.0

Bluefish, cooked, dry heat

3 oz (85g)	135	38	22	0	4	65	65	0.0

Burbot, cooked, dry heat

3 oz (85g)	98	8	21	0	1	65	105	0.0

Butterfish, cooked, dry heat

1 fillet (25g)	47	23	6	0	3	21	29	0.0

Carp, cooked, dry heat

3 oz (85g)	138	54	20	0	6	71	54	0.0

Catfish, channel, breaded and fried

3 oz (85g)	195	100	15	7	11	69	238	0.9

Catfish, channel, farmed, cooked, dry heat

3 oz (85g)	129	61	16	0	7	54	68	0.0

Catfish, channel, wild, cooked, dry heat

3 oz (85g)	89	23	15	0	3	61	43	0.0

Food Serving size	Cal.	Fat cal.	Prot.	Carb.	Fat	Chol.	Sod.	Fiber
Caviar, black and red, granular 1 tablespoon (16g)	40	26	4	1	3	94	240	0.0
Cisco, smoked 1 oz (28g)	50	30	4	0	3	9	135	0.0
Cod, Atlantic, canned, solids and liquid 3 oz (85g)	89	8	20	0	1	47	185	0.0
Cod, Atlantic, cooked, dry heat 3 oz (85g)	89	8	20	0	1	47	66	0.0
Cod, Atlantic, dried and salted 1 oz (28g)	81	5	18	0	1	43	1968	0.0
Cod, Pacific, cooked, dry heat 3 oz (85g)	89	8	20	0	1	40	77	0.0
Croaker, Atlantic, breaded and fried 3 oz (85g)	188	100	15	7	11	71	296	0.0
Cusk, cooked, dry heat 3 oz (85g)	95	8	20	0	1	45	34	0.0
Dolphinfish, cooked, dry heat 3 oz (85g)	93	8	20	0	1	80	96	0.0
Drum, freshwater, cooked, dry heat 3 oz (85g)	130	46	19	0	5	70	82	0.0
Eel, mixed species, cooked, dry heat 1 oz, with bone	52	30	5	0	3	35	14	0.0
Fish portions and sticks, frozen, preheated 1 stick (4"x 1"x $\frac{1}{2}$") (28g)	76	30	4	7	3	31	163	0.0
Flatfish (flounder and sole species), cooked, dry heat 3 oz (85g)	99	15	20	0	2	58	89	0.0
Gefiltefish, commercial, sweet recipe 1 piece (42g)	35	8	4	3	1	13	220	0.0
Grouper, mixed species, cooked, dry heat 3 oz (85g)	100	8	21	0	1	40	45	0.0
Haddock, cooked, dry heat 3 oz (85g)	95	8	20	0	1	63	74	0.0

Food Serving size	Cal.	Fat cal.	Prot.	Carb.	Fat	Chol.	Sod.	Fiber
Haddock, smoked 1 cubic inch, boneless (17g)	20	2	4	0	0	13	130	0.0
Halibut, Atlantic and Pacific, cooked, dry heat 3 oz (85g)	119	23	23	0	3	35	59	0.0
Halibut, greenland, cooked, dry heat 3 oz (85g)	203	138	15	0	15	50	88	0.0
Herring, Atlantic, cooked, dry heat 3 oz (85g)	173	92	20	0	10	65	98	0.0
Herring, Atlantic, kippered 1 cubic inch, boneless, cooked (17g)	37	18	4	0	2	14	156	0.0
Herring, Atlantic, pickled 1 oz, boneless (28g)	73	45	4	3	5	4	244	0.0
Herring, Pacific, cooked, dry heat 3 oz (85g)	213	138	18	0	15	84	81	0.0
Ling, cooked, dry heat 3 oz (85g)	94	8	20	0	1	43	147	0.0
Lingcod, cooked, dry heat 3 oz (85g)	93	8	20	0	1	57	65	0.0
Mackerel, Atlantic, cooked, dry heat 3 oz (85g)	223	138	20	0	15	64	71	0.0
Mackerel, jack, canned, drained solids 1 oz, boneless (28g)	44	15	6	0	2	22	106	0.0
Mackerel, king, cooked, dry heat 3 oz (85g)	114	23	22	0	3	58	173	0.0
Mackerel, Pacific and jack, mixed species, cooked, dry heat 1 cubic inch, boneless, cooked (17g)	34	15	4	0	2	10	19	0.0
Mackerel, Spanish, cooked, dry heat 3 oz (85g)	134	46	20	0	5	62	56	0.0
Milkfish, cooked, dry heat 3 oz (85g)	162	69	22	0	8	57	78	0.0
Monkfish, cooked, dry heat 3 oz (85g)	82	15	16	0	2	27	20	0.0

Food Serving size	Cal.	Fat cal.	Prot.	Carb.	Fat	Chol.	Sod.	Fiber
Mullet, striped, cooked, dry heat 3 oz (85g)	128	38	21	0	4	54	60	0.0
Ocean perch, Atlantic, cooked, dry heat 1 fillet (50g)	61	9	12	0	1	27	48	0.0
Perch, mixed species, cooked, dry heat 1 fillet (46g)	54	4	12	0	0	53	36	0.0
Pike, northern, cooked, dry heat 3 oz (85g)	96	8	21	0	1	43	42	0.0
Pike, walleye, cooked, dry heat 3 oz (85g)	101	15	21	0	2	94	55	0.0
Pollock, Atlantic, cooked, dry heat 3 oz (85g)	100	8	21	0	1	77	94	0.0
Pollock, walleye, cooked, dry heat 1 fillet (60g)	68	5	14	0	1	58	70	0.0
Pompano, Florida, cooked, dry heat 3 oz (85g)	179	92	20	0	10	54	65	0.0
Pout, ocean, cooked, dry heat 3 oz (85g)	87	8	18	0	1	57	66	0.0
Rockfish, Pacific, mixed species, cooked, dry heat 3 oz (85g)	103	15	20	0	2	37	65	0.0
Roe, mixed species, cooked, dry heat 1 oz (28g)	57	20	8	1	2	134	33	0.0
Roughy, orange, cooked, dry heat 3 oz (85g)	76	8	16	0	1	22	69	0.0
Sablefish, cooked, dry heat 3 oz (85g)	213	153	14	0	17	54	61	0.0
Sablefish, smoked 1 oz (28g)	72	51	5	0	6	18	206	0.0
Salmon, Atlantic, farmed, cooked, dry heat 3 oz (85g)	175	92	19	0	10	54	52	0.0
Salmon, Atlantic, wild, cooked, dry heat 3 oz (85g)	155	61	21	0	7	60	48	0.0
Salmon, chinook, cooked, dry heat 3 oz (85g)	196	100	22	0	11	72	51	0.0

Food

Serving size	Cal.	Fat cal.	Prot.	Carb.	Fat	Chol.	Sod.	Fiber
Salmon, chinook, smoked, (lox), regular								
1 oz (28g)	33	10	5	0	1	6	560	0.0
Salmon, chinook, smoked								
1 oz, boneless (28g)	33	10	5	0	1	6	220	0.0
Salmon, chum, canned, without salt, drained solids with bone								
3 oz (85g)	120	46	18	0	5	33	64	0.0
Salmon, chum, cooked, dry heat								
3 oz (85g)	131	38	22	0	4	81	54	0.0
Salmon, chum, drained solids with bone								
3 oz (85g)	120	46	18	0	5	33	414	0.0
Salmon, coho, farmed, cooked, dry heat								
3 oz (85g)	151	61	20	0	7	54	44	0.0
Salmon, coho, wild, cooked, dry heat								
3 oz (85g)	118	31	20	0	3	47	49	0.0
Salmon, coho, wild, cooked, moist heat								
3 oz (85g)	156	61	23	0	7	48	45	0.0
Salmon, pink, canned, solids with bone and liquid								
3 oz (85g)	118	46	17	0	5	47	471	0.0
Salmon, pink, canned, without salt, solids with bone and liquid								
3 oz (85g)	118	46	17	0	5	47	64	0.0
Salmon, pink, cooked, dry heat								
3 oz (85g)	127	31	22	0	3	57	73	0.0
Salmon, sockeye, canned, drained solids with bone								
3 oz (85g)	130	54	17	0	6	37	457	0.0
Salmon, sockeye, canned, without salt, drained solids with bone								
3 oz (85g)	130	54	17	0	6	37	64	0.0
Salmon, sockeye, cooked, dry heat								
3 oz (85g)	184	84	23	0	9	74	56	0.0
Sardine, Atlantic, canned in oil, drained solids with bone								
1 oz (28g)	58	28	7	0	3	40	141	0.0
Sardine, Pacific, canned in tomato sauce, drained solids with bone								
1 cup (89g)	158	96	14	0	11	54	368	0.0
Scup, cooked, dry heat								
1 fillet (50g)	68	18	12	0	2	34	27	0.0

Food Serving size	Cal.	Fat cal.	Prot.	Carb.	Fat	Chol.	Sod.	Fiber
Sea bass, mixed species, cooked, dry heat								
3 oz (85g)	105	23	20	0	3	45	74	0.0
Seatrout, mixed species, cooked, dry heat								
3 oz (85g)	113	38	18	0	4	90	63	0.0
Shad, american, cooked, dry heat								
3 oz (85g)	214	138	19	0	15	82	55	0.0
Shark, mixed species, batter-dipped and fried								
3 oz (85g)	194	107	16	5	12	50	104	0.0
Sheepshead, cooked, dry heat								
3 oz (85g)	107	15	22	0	2	54	62	0.0
Smelt, rainbow, cooked, dry heat								
3 oz (85g)	105	23	20	0	3	77	65	0.0
Snapper, mixed species, cooked, dry heat								
3 oz (85g)	109	15	22	0	2	40	48	0.0
Spot, cooked, dry heat								
1 fillet (50g)	79	27	12	0	3	39	19	0.0
Sturgeon, mixed species, cooked, dry heat 1 oz, boneless, cooked								
(28g)	38	13	6	0	1	22	19	0.0
Sturgeon, mixed species, smoked								
1 oz (28g)	48	10	9	0	1	22	207	0.0
Sucker, white, cooked, dry heat								
3 oz (85g)	101	23	18	0	3	45	43	0.0
Sunfish, pumpkin seed, cooked, dry heat								
1 fillet (37g)	42	3	9	0	0	32	38	0.0
Surimi								
1 oz (28g)	28	3	4	2	0	8	40	0.0
Swordfish, cooked, dry heat								
3 oz (85g)	132	38	21	0	4	43	98	0.0
Tilefish, cooked, dry heat								
3 oz (85g)	125	38	20	0	4	54	50	0.0
Trout, mixed species, cooked, dry heat								
1 fillet (62g)	118	45	17	0	5	46	42	0.0

Food Serving size	Cal.	Fat cal.	Prot.	Carb.	Fat	Chol.	Sod.	Fiber
Trout, rainbow, farmed, cooked, dry heat 1 fillet (71g)	120	45	17	0	5	48	30	0.0
Trout, rainbow, wild, cooked, dry heat 3 oz (85g)	128	46	20	0	5	59	48	0.0
Tuna salad 3 oz (85g)	159	69	14	8	8	11	342	0.0
Tuna, fresh, bluefin, cooked, dry heat 3 oz (85g)	156	46	26	0	5	42	43	0.0
Tuna, light, canned in oil, drained solids 1 oz (28g)	55	20	8	0	2	5	99	0.0
Tuna, light, canned in oil, without salt, drained solids 3 oz (85g)	168	61	25	0	7	15	43	0.0
Tuna, light, canned in water, drained solids 1 oz (28g)	32	3	7	0	0	8	95	0.0
Tuna, light, canned in water, without salt, drained solids 3 oz (85g)	99	8	22	0	1	26	43	0.0
Tuna, skipjack, fresh, cooked, dry heat 3 oz (85g)	112	8	24	0	1	51	40	0.0
Tuna, white, canned in oil, drained solids 3 oz (85g)	158	61	23	0	7	26	337	0.0
Tuna, white, canned in oil, without salt, drained solids 3 oz (85g)	158	61	23	0	7	26	43	0.0
Tuna, white, canned in water, drained solids 3 oz (85g)	109	23	20	0	3	36	320	0.0
Tuna, white, canned in water, without salt, drained solids 3 oz (85g)	109	23	20	0	3	36	43	0.0
Tuna, yellowfin, fresh, cooked, dry heat 3 oz (85g)	118	8	26	0	1	49	40	0.0
Turbot, European, cooked, dry heat 3 oz (85g)	104	31	18	0	3	53	163	0.0
Whitefish, mixed species, cooked, dry heat 3 oz (85g)	146	61	20	0	7	65	55	0.0
Whitefish, mixed species, smoked 1 oz, boneless (28g)	30	3	6	0	0	9	285	0.0

Food Serving size	Cal.	Fat cal.	Prot.	Carb.	Fat	Chol.	Sod.	Fiber
Whiting, mixed species, cooked, dry heat								
1 fillet (72g)	84	13	17	0	1	60	95	0.0
Wolffish, Atlantic, cooked, dry heat								
3 oz (85g)	105	23	19	0	3	50	93	0.0
Yellowtail, mixed species, cooked, dry heat								
3 oz (85g)	159	54	26	0	6	60	43	0.0

Shellfish

Food Serving size	Cal.	Fat cal.	Prot.	Carb.	Fat	Chol.	Sod.	Fiber
Crustaceans, crab, Alaska king, cooked, moist heat								
3 oz (85g)	82	15	16	0	2	45	911	0.0
Crustaceans, crab, Alaska king, imitation, made from surimi								
3 oz (85g)	87	8	10	9	1	17	715	0.0
Crustaceans, crab, blue, canned								
1 oz (28g)	28	3	6	0	0	25	93	0.0
Crustaceans, crab, blue, cooked, moist heat 1 cup, cooked, flaked								
and pieces (118g)	120	21	24	0	2	118	329	0.0
Crustaceans, crab, blue, crab cakes								
1 cake (60g)	93	42	12	0	5	90	198	0.0
Crustaceans, crab, Dungeness, cooked, moist heat								
3 oz (85g)	94	8	19	1	1	65	321	0.0
Crustaceans, crab, queen, cooked, moist heat								
3 oz (85g)	98	15	20	0	2	60	587	0.0
Crustaceans, crayfish, mixed species, farmed, cooked, moist heat								
3 oz (85g)	74	8	15	0	1	116	82	0.0
Crustaceans, crayfish, mixed species, wild, cooked, moist heat								
3 oz (85g)	70	8	14	0	1	113	80	0.0
Crustaceans, lobster, northern, cooked, moist heat								
3 oz (85g)	83	8	17	1	1	61	323	0.0
Crustaceans, shrimp, mixed species, breaded and fried								
4 large (30g)	73	32	6	3	4	53	103	0.0
Crustaceans, shrimp, mixed species, canned								
1 oz, cooked (28g)	34	5	6	0	1	48	47	0.0
Crustaceans, shrimp, mixed species, cooked, moist heat								
4 large (22g)	22	2	5	0	0	43	49	0.0

Food Serving size	Cal.	Fat cal.	Prot.	Carb.	Fat	Chol.	Sod.	Fiber
Crustaceans, shrimp, mixed species, imitation, made from surimi								
3 oz (85g)	86	8	10	8	1	31	599	0.0
Crustaceans, spiny lobster, mixed species, cooked, moist heat								
3 oz (85g)	122	15	22	3	2	77	193	0.0
Mollusks, abalone, mixed species, fried								
3 oz (85g)	161	53	17	9	6	80	502	0.0
Mollusks, clam, mixed species, breaded and fried								
3 oz (85g)	172	83	12	9	9	52	309	
Mollusks, clam, mixed species, canned, drained solids								
3 oz (85g)	126	15	22	4	2	57	95	0.0
Mollusks, clam, mixed species, canned, liquid								
3 oz (85g)	2	0	0	0	0	3	183	0.0
Mollusks, clam, mixed species, cooked, moist heat								
3 oz (85g)	126	15	22	4	2	57	95	0.0
Mollusks, cuttlefish, mixed species, cooked, moist heat								
3 oz (85g)	134	8	27	2	1	190	632	0.0
Mollusks, mussel, blue, cooked, moist heat								
3 oz (85g)	146	31	20	6	3	48	314	0.0
Mollusks, octopus, common, cooked, moist heat								
3 oz (85g)	139	15	26	3	2	82	391	0.0
Mollusks, oyster, eastern, breaded and fried								
3 oz (85g)	167	100	8	10	11	69	354	
Mollusks, oyster, eastern, canned								
1 cup, drained (162g)	112	29	11	6	3	89	181	0.0
Mollusks, oyster, eastern, farmed, cooked, dry heat								
6 medium (59g)	47	11	4	4	1	22	96	0.0
Mollusks, oyster, eastern, wild, cooked, dry heat								
6 medium (59g)	42	11	5	3	1	29	144	0.0
Mollusks, oyster, eastern, wild, cooked, moist heat								
6 medium (42g)	58	19	6	3	2	44	177	0.0
Mollusks, oyster, Pacific, cooked, moist heat								
1 medium (25g)	41	11	5	3	1	25	53	0.0
Mollusks, oyster, Pacific								
1 medium (50g)	41	9	5	3	1	25	53	0.0

Food Serving size	Cal.	Fat cal.	Prot.	Carb.	Fat	Chol.	Sod.	Fiber
Mollusks, scallop, mixed species, breaded and fried								
2 large scallops (31g)	67	30	6	3	3	19	144	
Mollusks, scallop, mixed species, imitation, made from surimi								
3 oz (85g)	84	0	11	9	0	19	676	0.0
Mollusks, squid, mixed species, fried								
3 oz (85g)	149	53	15	7	6	221	260	0.0
Mollusks, whelk, unspecified, cooked, moist heat								
3 oz (85g)	234	8	41	14	1	111	350	0.0

Lamb, Veal, and Game Products

Food Serving size	Cal.	Fat cal.	Prot.	Carb.	Fat	Chol.	Sod.	Fiber

Lamb

Lamb, domestic, composite of trimmed retail cuts, separable fat, trimmed to $\frac{1}{4}''$ fat, choice, cooked

3 oz (85g)	498	452	10	0	50	97	49	0.0

Lamb, domestic, composite of trimmed retail cuts, separable lean and fat, trimmed to $\frac{1}{8}''$ fat, choice, cooked

3 oz (85g)	230	138	22	0	15	82	61	0.0

Lamb, domestic, composite of trimmed retail cuts, separable lean and fat, trimmed to $\frac{1}{4}''$ fat, choice, cooked

3 oz (85g)	250	161	21	0	18	82	61	0.0

Lamb, domestic, composite of trimmed retail cuts, separable lean only, trimmed to $\frac{1}{4}''$ fat, choice, cooked

3 oz (85g)	175	77	24	0	9	78	65	0.0

Lamb, domestic, cubed for stew or kabob (leg and shoulder), separable lean only, trimmed to $\frac{1}{4}''$ fat, braised

3 oz (85g)	190	69	29	0	8	92	60	0.0

Lamb, domestic, cubed for stew or kabob (leg and shoulder), separable lean only, trimmed to $\frac{1}{4}''$ fat, broiled

3 oz (85g)	158	54	24	0	6	77	65	0.0

Lamb, domestic, foreshank, separable lean and fat, trimmed to $\frac{1}{8}''$ fat, braised

3 oz (85g)	207	100	24	0	11	90	61	0.0

Food Serving size	Cal.	Fat cal.	Prot.	Carb.	Fat	Chol.	Sod.	Fiber
Lamb, domestic, foreshank, separable lean and fat, trimmed to $\frac{1}{4}$" fat, choice, braised								
3 oz (85g)	207	100	24	0	11	90	61	0.0
Lamb, domestic, foreshank, separable lean only, trimmed to $\frac{1}{4}$" fat, choice, braised								
3 oz (85g)	159	46	26	0	5	88	63	0.0
Lamb, domestic, leg, shank half, separable lean and fat, trimmed to $\frac{1}{8}$" fat, choice, roasted								
3 oz (85g)	184	84	23	0	9	77	55	0.0
Lamb, domestic, leg, shank half, separable lean and fat, trimmed to $\frac{1}{4}$" fat, choice, roasted								
3 oz (85g)	191	92	22	0	10	77	55	0.0
Lamb, domestic, leg, shank half, separable lean only, trimmed to $\frac{1}{4}$" fat, choice, roasted								
3 oz (85g)	153	54	24	0	6	74	56	0.0
Lamb, domestic, leg, sirloin half, separable lean and fat, trimmed to $\frac{1}{8}$" fat, choice, roasted								
3 oz (85g)	241	153	21	0	17	82	58	0.0
Lamb, domestic, leg, sirloin half, separable lean and fat, trimmed to $\frac{1}{4}$" fat, choice, roasted								
3 oz (85g)	248	161	21	0	18	82	58	0.0
Lamb, domestic, leg, sirloin half, separable lean only, trimmed to $\frac{1}{4}$" fat, choice, roasted								
3 oz (85g)	173	69	24	0	8	78	60	0.0
Lamb, domestic, leg, whole (shank and sirloin), separable lean and fat, trimmed to $\frac{1}{8}$" fat, choice, roasted								
3 oz (85g)	206	107	22	0	12	78	57	0.0
Lamb, domestic, leg, whole (shank and sirloin), separable lean and fat, trimmed to $\frac{1}{4}$" fat, choice, roasted								
3 oz (85g)	219	123	22	0	14	79	56	0.0
Lamb, domestic, leg, whole (shank and sirloin), separable lean only, trimmed to $\frac{1}{4}$" fat, choice, roasted								
3 oz (85g)	162	61	24	0	7	76	58	0.0
Lamb, domestic, loin, separable lean and fat, trimmed to $\frac{1}{8}$" fat, choice, broiled								
1 raw steak with refuse, (102 g)	157	100	14	0	11	52	41	0.0

Food
Serving size	Cal.	Fat cal.	Prot.	Carb.	Fat	Chol.	Sod.	Fiber
Lamb, domestic, loin, separable lean and fat, trimmed to $\frac{1}{8}''$ fat, choice, roasted							
3 oz (85g)	247	161	20	0	18	79	54	0.0
Lamb, domestic, loin, separable lean and fat, trimmed to $\frac{1}{4}''$ fat, choice, broiled							
1 raw chop with refuse							
(120 g)	202	133	16	0	15	64	49	0.0
Lamb, domestic, loin, separable lean and fat, trimmed to $\frac{1}{4}''$ fat, choice, roasted							
3 oz (85g)	263	184	20	0	20	81	54	0.0
Lamb, domestic, loin, separable lean only, trimmed to $\frac{1}{4}''$ fat, choice, broiled							
1 raw chop with refuse,							
(120 g)	99	41	14	0	5	44	39	0.0
Lamb, domestic, loin, separable lean only, trimmed to $\frac{1}{4}''$ fat, choice, roasted							
3 oz (85g)	172	77	23	0	9	74	56	0.0
Lamb, domestic, rib, separable lean and fat, trimmed to $\frac{1}{8}''$ fat, choice, broiled							
3 oz (85g)	289	207	20	0	23	83	65	0.0
Lamb, domestic, rib, separable lean and fat, trimmed to $\frac{1}{8}''$ fat, choice, roasted							
3 oz (85g)	290	215	19	0	24	82	63	0.0
Lamb, domestic, rib, separable lean and fat, trimmed to $\frac{1}{4}''$ fat, choice, broiled							
3 oz (85g)	307	230	19	0	26	84	65	0.0
Lamb, domestic, rib, separable lean and fat, trimmed to $\frac{1}{4}''$ fat, choice, roasted							
3 oz (85g)	305	230	18	0	26	82	62	0.0
Lamb, domestic, rib, separable lean only, trimmed to $\frac{1}{4}''$ fat, choice, broiled							
3 oz (85g)	200	100	24	0	11	77	72	0.0
Lamb, domestic, rib, separable lean only, trimmed to $\frac{1}{4}''$ fat, choice, roasted							
3 oz (85g)	197	100	22	0	11	75	69	0.0

Food Serving size	Cal.	Fat cal.	Prot.	Carb.	Fat	Chol.	Sod.	Fiber
Lamb, domestic, shoulder, arm, separable lean and fat, trimmed to $\frac{1}{8}$″ fat, broiled 1 raw steak with refuse, (102 g)	159	96	15	0	11	57	46	0.0
Lamb, domestic, shoulder, arm, separable lean and fat, trimmed to $\frac{1}{8}$″ fat, choice, braised 1 raw steak with refuse, (102 g)	152	93	14	0	10	54	32	0.0
Lamb, domestic, shoulder, arm, separable lean and fat, trimmed to $\frac{1}{8}$″ fat, choice, roasted 3 oz (85g)	227	146	20	0	16	77	55	0.0
Lamb, domestic, shoulder, arm, separable lean and fat, trimmed to $\frac{1}{4}$″ fat, choice, braised 1 raw chop with refuse, (160 g)	242	152	21	0	17	84	50	0.0
Lamb, domestic, shoulder, arm, separable lean and fat, trimmed to $\frac{1}{4}$″ fat, choice, broiled 3 oz (85g)	239	153	20	0	17	82	65	0.0
Lamb, domestic, shoulder, arm, separable lean and fat, trimmed to $\frac{1}{4}$″ fat, choice, roasted 3 oz (85g)	237	153	20	0	17	78	55	0.0
Lamb, domestic, shoulder, arm, separable lean only, trimmed to $\frac{1}{4}$″ fat, choice, braised 1 raw chop with refuse, (160 g)	153	69	20	0	8	67	42	0.0
Lamb, domestic, shoulder, arm, separable lean only, trimmed to $\frac{1}{4}$″ fat, choice, broiled 1 raw chop with refuse, (160 g)	148	60	21	0	7	68	61	0.0
Lamb, domestic, shoulder, arm, separable lean only, trimmed to $\frac{1}{4}$″ fat, choice, roasted 3 oz (85g)	163	69	21	0	8	73	57	0.0
Lamb, domestic, shoulder, blade, separable lean and fat, trimmed to $\frac{1}{4}$″ fat, choice, braised 3 oz (85g)	288	184	25	0	20	99	64	0.0
Lamb, domestic, shoulder, blade, separable lean and fat, trimmed to $\frac{1}{8}$″ fat, choice, broiled 3 oz (85g)	227	138	20	0	15	81	71	0.0

Food
Serving size | Cal. | Fat cal. | Prot. | Carb. | Fat | Chol. | Sod. | Fiber

Food / Serving size	Cal.	Fat cal.	Prot.	Carb.	Fat	Chol.	Sod.	Fiber
Lamb, domestic, shoulder, blade, separable lean and fat, trimmed to $\frac{1}{8}''$ fat, choice, roasted								
3 oz (85g)	230	146	20	0	16	78	57	0.0
Lamb, domestic, shoulder, blade, separable lean and fat, trimmed to $\frac{1}{4}''$ fat, choice, braised								
3 oz (85g)	293	192	25	0	21	99	64	0.0
Lamb, domestic, shoulder, blade, separable lean and fat, trimmed to $\frac{1}{4}''$ fat, choice, broiled								
3 oz (85g)	236	153	20	0	17	81	70	0.0
Lamb, domestic, shoulder, blade, separable lean and fat, trimmed to $\frac{1}{4}''$ fat, choice, roasted								
3 oz (85g)	239	161	19	0	18	78	56	0.0
Lamb, domestic, shoulder, blade, separable lean only, trimmed to $\frac{1}{4}''$ fat, choice, braised								
3 oz (85g)	245	130	27	0	14	99	67	0.0
Lamb, domestic, shoulder, blade, separable lean only, trimmed to $\frac{1}{4}''$ fat, choice, broiled								
3 oz (85g)	179	84	21	0	9	77	75	0.0
Lamb, domestic, shoulder, blade, separable lean only, trimmed to $\frac{1}{4}''$ fat, choice, roasted								
3 oz (85g)	178	92	21	0	10	74	58	0.0
Lamb, domestic, shoulder, whole (arm and blade), separable lean and fat, trimmed to $\frac{1}{8}''$ fat, choice, braised								
3 oz (85g)	287	184	25	0	20	99	63	0.0
Lamb, domestic, shoulder, whole (arm and blade), separable lean and fat, trimmed to $\frac{1}{8}''$ fat, choice, broiled								
3 oz (85g)	228	138	20	0	15	81	70	0.0
Lamb, domestic, shoulder, whole (arm and blade), separable lean and fat, trimmed to $\frac{1}{8}''$ fat, choice, roasted								
3 oz (85g)	229	146	20	0	16	77	56	0.0
Lamb, domestic, shoulder, whole (arm and blade), separable lean and fat, trimmed to $\frac{1}{4}''$ fat, choice, braised								
3 oz (85g)	292	192	25	0	21	99	64	0.0
Lamb, domestic, shoulder, whole (arm and blade), separable lean and fat, trimmed to $\frac{1}{4}''$ fat, choice, broiled								
3 oz (85g)	236	146	20	0	16	82	66	0.0

Food Serving size	Cal.	Fat cal.	Prot.	Carb.	Fat	Chol.	Sod.	Fiber
Lamb, domestic, shoulder, whole (arm and blade), separable lean and fat, trimmed to $\frac{1}{4}''$ fat, choice, roasted								
3 oz (85g)	235	153	20	0	17	78	56	0.0
Lamb, domestic, shoulder, whole (arm and blade), separable lean only, trimmed to $\frac{1}{4}''$ fat, choice, braised								
3 oz (85g)	241	123	28	0	14	99	67	0.0
Lamb, domestic, shoulder, whole (arm and blade), separable lean only, trimmed to $\frac{1}{4}''$ fat, choice, broiled								
3 oz (85g)	179	77	23	0	9	79	71	0.0
Lamb, domestic, shoulder, whole (arm and blade), separable lean only, trimmed to $\frac{1}{4}''$ fat, choice, roasted								
3 oz (85g)	173	84	21	0	9	74	58	0.0
Lamb, ground, broiled								
3 oz (85g)	241	153	21	0	17	82	69	0.0
Lamb, New Zealand, imported, frozen, composite of trimmed retail cuts, separable fat, cooked								
3 oz (85g)	498	460	9	0	51	93	30	0.0
Lamb, New Zealand, imported, frozen, composite of trimmed retail cuts, separable lean and fat, cooked								
3 oz (85g)	259	169	20	0	19	93	39	0.0
Lamb, New Zealand, imported, frozen, composite of trimmed retail cuts, separable lean and fat, trimmed to $\frac{1}{8}''$ fat, cooked								
3 oz (85g)	230	138	21	0	15	90	39	0.0
Lamb, New Zealand, imported, frozen, composite of trimmed retail cuts, separable lean only, cooked								
3 oz (85g)	175	69	26	0	8	93	43	0.0
Lamb, New Zealand, imported, frozen, foreshank, separable lean and fat, braised								
3 oz (85g)	219	123	23	0	14	87	40	0.0
Lamb, New Zealand, imported, frozen, foreshank, separable lean and fat, trimmed to $\frac{1}{8}''$ fat, braised								
3 oz (85g)	219	123	23	0	14	87	40	0.0
Lamb, New Zealand, imported, frozen, foreshank, separable lean only, braised								
3 oz (85g)	158	46	26	0	5	86	42	0.0

Food
Serving size	Cal.	Fat cal.	Prot.	Carb.	Fat	Chol.	Sod.	Fiber

Lamb, New Zealand, imported, frozen, leg, whole (shank and sirloin), separable lean and fat, roasted
| 3 oz (85g) | 209 | 123 | 21 | 0 | 14 | 86 | 37 | 0.0 |

Lamb, New Zealand, imported, frozen, leg, whole (shank and sirloin), separable lean and fat, trimmed to $\frac{1}{8}''$ fat, roasted
| 3 oz (85g) | 199 | 107 | 21 | 0 | 12 | 86 | 37 | 0.0 |

Lamb, New Zealand, imported, frozen, leg, whole (shank and sirloin), separable lean only, roasted
| 3 oz (85g) | 154 | 54 | 24 | 0 | 6 | 85 | 38 | 0.0 |

Lamb, New Zealand, imported, frozen, loin, separable lean and fat, broiled
1 raw chop with refuse,
| (85 g) | 135 | 93 | 10 | 0 | 10 | 48 | 21 | 0.0 |

Lamb, New Zealand, imported, frozen, loin, separable lean and fat, trimmed to $\frac{1}{8}''$ fat, broiled
1 raw chop with refuse,
| (85 g) | 124 | 80 | 10 | 0 | 9 | 47 | 21 | 0.0 |

Lamb, New Zealand, imported, frozen, loin, separable lean only, broiled
1 raw chop with refuse,
| (85 g) | 60 | 22 | 9 | 0 | 2 | 34 | 17 | 0.0 |

Lamb, New Zealand, imported, frozen, rib, separable lean and fat, roasted
| 3 oz (85g) | 289 | 222 | 16 | 0 | 25 | 85 | 37 | 0.0 |

Lamb, New Zealand, imported, frozen, rib, separable lean and fat, trimmed to $\frac{1}{8}''$ fat, roasted
| 3 oz (85g) | 269 | 199 | 17 | 0 | 22 | 84 | 37 | 0.0 |

Lamb, New Zealand, imported, frozen, rib, separable lean, roasted
| 3 oz (85g) | 167 | 77 | 20 | 0 | 9 | 80 | 41 | 0.0 |

Lamb, New Zealand, imported, frozen, shoulder, whole (arm and blade), separable lean and fat, braised
| 3 oz (85g) | 303 | 199 | 24 | 0 | 22 | 105 | 43 | 0.0 |

Lamb, New Zealand, imported, frozen, shoulder, whole (arm and blade), separable lean and fat, trimmed to $\frac{1}{8}''$ fat, braised
| 3 oz (85g) | 291 | 184 | 25 | 0 | 20 | 105 | 44 | 0.0 |

Lamb, New Zealand, imported, frozen, shoulder, whole (arm and blade), separable lean only, braised
| 3 oz (85g) | 242 | 123 | 29 | 0 | 14 | 108 | 48 | 0.0 |

Food Serving size	Cal.	Fat cal.	Prot.	Carb.	Fat	Chol.	Sod.	Fiber
Lamb, variety meats and by-products, kidneys, braised								
3 oz (85g)	116	31	20	1	3	480	128	0.0
Lamb, variety meats and by-products, liver, braised								
3 oz (85g)	187	69	26	3	8	426	48	0.0
Lamb, variety meats and by-products, liver, pan-fried								
3 oz (85g)	202	100	22	3	11	419	105	0.0
Lamb, variety meats and by-products, lungs, braised								
3 oz (85g)	96	23	17	0	3	241	71	0.0
Lamb, variety meats and by-products, pancreas, braised								
3 oz (85g)	199	115	20	0	13	340	44	0.0
Lamb, variety meats and by-products, tongue, braised								
3 oz (85g)	234	153	19	0	17	161	57	0.0

Veal

Food Serving size	Cal.	Fat cal.	Prot.	Carb.	Fat	Chol.	Sod.	Fiber
Veal, breast, plate half, boneless, separable lean and fat, braised								
3 oz (85g)	240	146	22	0	16	95	54	
Veal, breast, point half, boneless, separable lean and fat, braised								
3 oz (85g)	211	107	24	0	12	97	56	
Veal, breast, separable fat, cooked								
1 oz (28g)	146	134	3	0	15	27	14	0.0
Veal, breast, whole, boneless, separable lean and fat, braised								
3 oz (85g)	226	130	23	0	14	96	55	
Veal, breast, whole, boneless, separable lean only, braised								
3 oz (85g)	185	77	26	0	9	99	58	
Veal, composite of trimmed retail cuts, separable fat, cooked								
3 oz (85g)	546	514	8	0	57	62	48	0.0
Veal, composite of trimmed retail cuts, separable lean and fat, cooked								
3 oz (85g)	196	84	26	0	9	97	74	0.0
Veal, composite of trimmed retail cuts, separable lean only, cooked								
3 oz (85g)	167	54	27	0	6	100	76	0.0
Veal, cubed for stew (leg and shoulder), separable lean only, braised								
3 oz (85g)	160	31	30	0	3	123	79	0.0
Veal, ground, broiled								
3 oz (85g)	146	61	20	0	7	88	71	0.0

Food Serving size	Cal.	Fat cal.	Prot.	Carb.	Fat	Chol.	Sod.	Fiber
Veal, leg (top round), separable lean and fat, braised 3 oz (85g)	179	46	31	0	5	114	57	0.0
Veal, leg (top round), separable lean and fat, pan-fried, breaded 3 oz (85g)	194	69	23	9	8	95	386	0.0
Veal, leg (top round), separable lean and fat, pan-fried, not breaded 3 oz (85g)	179	61	27	0	7	89	65	0.0
Veal, leg (top round), separable lean and fat, roasted 3 oz (85g)	136	38	24	0	4	88	58	0.0
Veal, leg (top round), separable lean only, braised 3 oz (85g)	173	38	31	0	4	115	57	0.0
Veal, leg (top round), separable lean only, pan-fried, breaded 3 oz (85g)	175	46	24	9	5	96	387	0.0
Veal, leg (top round), separable lean only, pan-fried, not breaded 3 oz (85g)	156	38	28	0	4	91	65	0.0
Veal, leg (top round), separable lean only, roasted 3 oz (85g)	128	23	24	0	3	88	58	0.0
Veal, loin, separable lean and fat, braised 1 raw chop with refuse, (195 g)	227	123	24	0	14	94	64	0.0
Veal, loin, separable lean and fat, roasted 3 oz (85g)	184	92	21	0	10	88	79	0.0
Veal, loin, separable lean only, braised 1 raw chop with refuse, (195 g)	156	56	23	0	6	86	58	0.0
Veal, loin, separable lean only, roasted 3 oz (85g)	149	54	22	0	6	90	82	0.0
Veal, rib, separable lean and fat, braised 3 oz (85g)	213	100	27	0	11	118	81	0.0
Veal, rib, separable lean and fat, roasted 3 oz (85g)	194	107	20	0	12	94	78	0.0
Veal, rib, separable lean only, braised 3 oz (85g)	185	61	29	0	7	122	84	0.0
Veal, rib, separable lean only, roasted 3 oz (85g)	150	54	22	0	6	98	82	0.0

Food Serving size	Cal.	Fat cal.	Prot.	Carb.	Fat	Chol.	Sod.	Fiber
Veal, shank (fore and hind), separable lean and fat, braised								
3 oz (85g)	162	46	27	0	5	105	79	
Veal, shank (fore and hind), separable lean only, braised								
3 oz (85g)	150	31	27	0	3	107	80	0.0
Veal, shoulder, arm, separable lean and fat, braised								
3 oz (85g)	201	77	29	0	9	126	74	0.0
Veal, shoulder, arm, separable lean and fat, roasted								
3 oz (85g)	156	61	21	0	7	92	77	0.0
Veal, shoulder, arm, separable lean only, braised								
3 oz (85g)	171	38	31	0	4	132	77	0.0
Veal, shoulder, arm, separable lean only, roasted								
3 oz (85g)	139	46	22	0	5	93	77	0.0
Veal, shoulder, blade, separable lean and fat, braised								
3 oz (85g)	191	77	26	0	9	130	83	0.0
Veal, shoulder, blade, separable lean and fat, roasted								
3 oz (85g)	158	69	21	0	8	99	85	0.0
Veal, shoulder, blade, separable lean only, braised								
3 oz (85g)	168	46	28	0	5	134	86	0.0
Veal, shoulder, blade, separable lean only, roasted								
3 oz (85g)	145	54	22	0	6	101	87	0.0
Veal, shoulder, whole (arm and blade), separable lean and fat, braised								
3 oz (85g)	194	77	27	0	9	107	81	0.0
Veal, shoulder, whole (arm and blade), separable lean and fat, roasted								
3 oz (85g)	156	61	21	0	7	96	82	0.0
Veal, shoulder, whole (arm and blade), separable lean only, braised								
3 oz (85g)	169	46	29	0	5	111	82	0.0
Veal, shoulder, whole (arm and blade), separable lean only, roasted								
3 oz (85g)	145	54	22	0	6	97	82	0.0
Veal, sirloin, separable lean and fat, braised								
3 oz (85g)	214	100	26	0	11	92	67	0.0
Veal, sirloin, separable lean and fat, roasted								
3 oz (85g)	172	77	21	0	9	87	71	0.0
Veal, sirloin, separable lean only, braised								
3 oz (85g)	173	54	29	0	6	96	69	0.0

Food Serving size	Cal.	Fat cal.	Prot.	Carb.	Fat	Chol.	Sod.	Fiber
Veal, sirloin, separable lean only, roasted								
3 oz (85g)	143	46	22	0	5	88	72	0.0
Veal, variety meats and by-products, liver, braised								
3 oz (85g)	140	54	19	3	6	477	45	0.0
Veal, variety meats and by-products, liver, pan-fried								
3 oz (85g)	208	84	26	3	9	281	112	0.0
Veal, variety meats and by-products, lungs, braised								
3 oz (85g)	88	23	16	0	3	224	48	0.0
Veal, variety meats and by-products, pancreas, braised								
3 oz (85g)	218	115	25	0	13		58	0.0

Game

Food Serving size	Cal.	Fat cal.	Prot.	Carb.	Fat	Chol.	Sod.	Fiber
Game meat, antelope, roasted								
3 oz (85g)	128	23	25	0	3	107	46	0.0
Game meat, bear, simmered								
3 oz (85g)	220	100	27	0	11	83	60	0.0
Game meat, beefalo, composite of cuts, roasted								
3 oz (85g)	160	46	26	0	5	49	70	0.0
Game meat, bison, roasted								
3 oz (85g)	122	15	24	0	2	70	48	0.0
Game meat, boar, wild, roasted								
3 oz (85g)	136	31	24	0	3	65	51	0.0
Game meat, caribou, roasted								
3 oz (85g)	142	31	26	0	3	93	51	0.0
Game meat, deer, roasted								
3 oz (85g)	134	23	26	0	3	95	46	0.0
Game meat, elk, roasted								
3 oz (85g)	124	15	26	0	2	62	52	0.0
Game meat, goat, roasted								
3 oz (85g)	122	23	23	0	3	64	73	0.0
Game meat, moose, roasted								
3 oz (85g)	114	8	25	0	1	66	59	0.0
Game meat, rabbit, domesticated, composite of cuts, roasted								
3 oz (85g)	167	61	25	0	7	70	40	0.0

Food Serving size	Cal.	Fat cal.	Prot.	Carb.	Fat	Chol.	Sod.	Fiber
Game meat, rabbit, domesticated, composite of cuts, stewed								
3 oz (85g)	175	61	26	0	7	73	31	0.0
Game meat, rabbit, wild, stewed								
3 oz (85g)	147	31	28	0	3	105	38	0.0
Game meat, raccoon, roasted								
3 oz (85g)	217	107	25	0	12	82	67	0.0
Game meat, squirrel, roasted								
3 oz (85g)	147	38	26	0	4	103	101	0.0

Pork Products

Food Serving size	Cal.	Fat cal.	Prot.	Carb.	Fat	Chol.	Sod.	Fiber

Fresh Pork

Pork, fresh, backribs, separable lean and fat, roasted

3 oz (85g)	315	230	20	0	26	100	86	0.0

Pork, fresh, composite of trimmed retail cuts (leg, loin, and shoulder), separable lean only, cooked

3 oz (85g)	180	77	25	0	9	73	50	0.0

Pork, fresh, composite of trimmed retail cuts (leg, loin, shoulder, and spareribs), separable lean and fat, cooked

3 oz (85g)	232	130	24	0	14	77	53	0.0

Pork, fresh, composite of trimmed retail cuts (loin and shoulder blade), separable lean and fat, cooked

3 oz (85g)	214	115	24	0	13	73	48	0.0

Pork, fresh, composite of trimmed retail cuts (loin and shoulder blade), separable lean only, cooked

3 oz (85g)	179	69	25	0	8	72	48	0.0

Pork, fresh, ground, cooked

3 oz (85g)	252	161	22	0	18	80	62	0.0

Pork, fresh, leg (ham), rump half, separable lean and fat, roasted

3 oz (85g)	214	107	25	0	12	82	53	0.0

Pork, fresh, leg (ham), rump half, separable lean only, roasted

3 oz (85g)	175	61	26	0	7	82	55	0.0

Pork, fresh, leg (ham), shank half, separable lean and fat, roasted

3 oz (85g)	246	153	21	0	17	78	50	0.0

Pork, fresh, leg (ham), shank half, separable lean only, roasted

3 oz (85g)	183	77	24	0	9	78	54	0.0

Food Serving size	Cal.	Fat cal.	Prot.	Carb.	Fat	Chol.	Sod.	Fiber
Pork, fresh, leg (ham), whole, separable lean only, roasted 3 oz (85g)	179	69	25	0	8	80	54	0.0
Pork, fresh, loin, blade (chops), bone-in, separable lean and fat, braised 1 raw chop with refuse, (151 g)	268	187	18	0	21	71	46	0.0
Pork, fresh, loin, blade (chops), bone-in, separable lean and fat, broiled 1 raw chop with refuse, (151 g)	256	180	18	0	20	69	56	0.0
Pork, fresh, loin, blade (chops), bone-in, separable lean and fat, pan-fried 1 raw chop with refuse, (151 g)	284	210	17	0	23	71	56	0.0
Pork, fresh, loin, blade (chops), bone-in, separable lean only, braised 1 raw chop with refuse, (151 g)	142	74	16	0	8	52	39	0.0
Pork, fresh, loin, blade (chops), bone-in, separable lean only, broiled 1 raw chop with refuse, (151 g)	147	80	16	0	9	53	50	0.0
Pork, fresh, loin, blade (chops), bone-in, separable lean only, pan-fried 1 raw chop with refuse, (151 g)	152	85	16	0	9	52	49	0.0
Pork, fresh, loin, blade (roasts), bone-in, separable lean and fat, roasted 3 oz (85g)	275	192	20	0	21	79	26	0.0
Pork, fresh, loin, blade (roasts), bone-in, separable lean only, roasted 3 oz (85g)	210	115	23	0	13	79	25	0.0
Pork, fresh, loin, center loin (chops), bone-in, separable lean and fat, braised 1 raw chop with refuse, (151 g)	205	105	23	0	12	71	49	0.0
Pork, fresh, loin, center loin (chops), bone-in, separable lean and fat, broiled 1 raw chop with refuse, (151 g)	197	96	24	0	11	67	48	0.0

Food Serving size	Cal.	Fat cal.	Prot.	Carb.	Fat	Chol.	Sod.	Fiber
Pork, fresh, loin, center loin (chops), bone-in, separable lean and fat, pan-fried 1 raw chop with refuse, (151 g)	216	120	23	0	13	72	62	0.0
Pork, fresh, loin, center loin (chops), bone-in, separable lean only, braised 1 raw chop with refuse, (151 g)	149	53	22	0	6	63	46	0.0
Pork, fresh, loin, center loin (chops), bone-in, separable lean only, broiled 1 raw chop with refuse, (151 g)	149	53	22	0	6	61	44	0.0
Pork, fresh, loin, center loin (chops), bone-in, separable lean only, pan-fried 1 raw chop with refuse, (151 g)	160	62	22	0	7	63	59	0.0
Pork, fresh, loin, center loin (roasts), bone-in, separable lean and fat, roasted 3 oz (85g)	199	100	22	0	11	68	54	0.0
Pork, fresh, loin, center loin (roasts), bone-in, separable lean only, roasted 3 oz (85g)	169	69	24	0	8	67	56	0.0
Pork, fresh, loin, center rib (chops), bone-in, separable lean and fat, braised 1 raw chop with refuse, (151 g)	188	101	20	0	11	55	30	0.0
Pork, fresh, loin, center rib (chops), bone-in, separable lean and fat, broiled 1 raw chop with refuse, (151 g)	195	100	21	0	11	61	46	0.0
Pork, fresh, loin, center rib (chops), bone-in, separable lean and fat, pan-fried 1 raw chop with refuse, (151 g)	193	112	19	0	12	53	37	0.0
Pork, fresh, loin, center rib (chops), bone-in, separable lean only, braised 1 raw chop with refuse, (151 g)	138	54	19	0	6	48	27	0.0

Food Serving size	Cal.	Fat cal.	Prot.	Carb.	Fat	Chol.	Sod.	Fiber
Pork, fresh, loin, center rib (chops), bone-in, separable lean only, broiled								
1 raw chop with refuse, (151 g)	147	60	21	0	7	54	44	0.0
Pork, fresh, loin, center rib (chops), bone-in, separable lean only, pan-fried								
1 raw chop with refuse, (151 g)	140	64	18	0	7	45	33	0.0
Pork, fresh, loin, center rib (chops), boneless, separable lean and fat, braised								
1 raw chop with refuse, (113 g)	207	117	21	0	13	59	32	0.0
Pork, fresh, loin, center rib (chops), boneless, separable lean and fat, broiled								
1 raw chop with refuse, (113 g)	208	115	22	0	13	66	50	0.0
Pork, fresh, loin, center rib (chops), boneless, separable lean and fat, pan-fried								
1 raw chop with refuse, (113 g)	168	81	21	0	9	53	39	0.0
Pork, fresh, loin, center rib (chops), boneless, separable lean only, braised								
1 raw chop with refuse, (113 g)	152	65	20	0	7	51	30	0.0
Pork, fresh, loin, center rib (chops), boneless, separable lean only, broiled								
1 raw chop with refuse, (113 g)	153	64	21	0	7	58	46	0.0
Pork, fresh, loin, center rib (chops), boneless, separable lean only, pan-fried								
1 raw chop with refuse, (113 g)	148	71	18	0	8	46	34	0.0
Pork, fresh, loin, center rib (roasts), bone-in, separable lean and fat, roasted								
3 oz (85g)	217	115	23	0	13	62	39	0.0
Pork, fresh, loin, center rib (roasts), bone-in, separable lean only, roasted								
3 oz (85g)	190	84	25	0	9	60	40	0.0

Food Serving size	Cal.	Fat cal.	Prot.	Carb.	Fat	Chol.	Sod.	Fiber
Pork, fresh, loin, center rib (roasts), boneless, separable lean and fat, roasted								
3 oz (85g)	214	115	23	0	13	69	41	0.0
Pork, fresh, loin, center rib (roasts), boneless, separable lean only, roasted								
3 oz (85g)	182	77	25	0	9	71	43	0.0
Pork, fresh, loin, country-style ribs, separable lean and fat, braised								
3 oz (85g)	252	169	20	0	19	74	50	0.0
Pork, fresh, loin, country-style ribs, separable lean and fat, roasted								
3 oz (85g)	279	192	20	0	21	78	44	0.0
Pork, fresh, loin, country-style ribs, separable lean only, braised								
3 oz (85g)	199	107	22	0	12	73	54	0.0
Pork, fresh, loin, country-style ribs, separable lean only, roasted								
3 oz (85g)	210	115	23	0	13	79	25	0.0
Pork, fresh, loin, sirloin (chops), bone-in, separable lean and fat, braised 1 raw chop with refuse,								
(151 g)	196	108	20	0	12	66	41	0.0
Pork, fresh, loin, sirloin (chops), bone-in, separable lean and fat, broiled 1 raw chop with refuse,								
(151 g)	194	108	20	0	12	65	51	0.0
Pork, fresh, loin, sirloin (chops), bone-in, separable lean only, braised 1 raw chop with refuse,								
(151 g)	142	58	19	0	6	58	38	0.0
Pork, fresh, loin, sirloin (chops), bone-in, separable lean only, broiled 1 raw chop with refuse,								
(151 g)	143	60	19	0	7	57	48	0.0
Pork, fresh, loin, sirloin (chops), boneless, separable lean and fat, braised 1 raw chop with refuse,								
(113 g)	155	59	22	0	7	66	38	0.0
Pork, fresh, loin, sirloin (chops), boneless, separable lean and fat, broiled 1 raw chop with refuse,								
(113 g)	154	60	23	0	7	67	41	0.0

Food Serving size	Cal.	Fat cal.	Prot.	Carb.	Fat	Chol.	Sod.	Fiber
Pork, fresh, loin, sirloin (chops), boneless, separable lean only, braised 1 raw chop with refuse, (113 g)	140	51	22	0	6	65	37	0.0
Pork, fresh, loin, sirloin (chops), boneless, separable lean only, broiled 1 raw chop with refuse, (113 g)	137	45	22	0	5	65	40	0.0
Pork, fresh, loin, sirloin (roasts), bone-in, separable lean and fat, roasted 3 oz (85g)	222	123	23	0	14	74	51	0.0
Pork, fresh, loin, sirloin (roasts), bone-in, separable lean only, roasted 3 oz (85g)	184	77	25	0	9	73	54	0.0
Pork, fresh, loin, sirloin (roasts), boneless, separable lean and fat, roasted 3 oz (85g)	176	69	24	0	8	73	48	0.0
Pork, fresh, loin, sirloin (roasts), boneless, separable lean only, roasted 3 oz (85g)	168	61	25	0	7	73	48	0.0
Pork, fresh, loin, tenderloin, separable lean and fat, broiled 1 raw chop with refuse, (113 g)	153	55	23	0	6	71	49	0.0
Pork, fresh, loin, tenderloin, separable lean and fat, roasted 3 oz (85g)	147	46	24	0	5	67	47	0.0
Pork, fresh, loin, tenderloin, separable lean only, broiled 1 raw chop with refuse, (113 g)	137	40	22	0	4	69	47	0.0
Pork, fresh, loin, tenderloin, separable lean only, roasted 3 oz (85g)	139	38	24	0	4	67	48	0.0
Pork, fresh, loin, top loin (chops), boneless, separable lean and fat, braised 1 lb raw with refuse	184	93	22	0	10	59	33	0.0
Pork, fresh, loin, top loin (chops), boneless, separable lean and fat, broiled 1 raw chop with refuse, (113 g)	163	70	21	0	8	58	45	0.0
Pork, fresh, loin, top loin (chops), boneless, separable lean and fat, pan-fried 1 raw chop with refuse, (113 g)	177	93	20	0	10	54	38	0.0

Food Serving size	Cal.	Fat cal.	Prot.	Carb.	Fat	Chol.	Sod.	Fiber
Pork, fresh, loin, top loin (chops), boneless, separable lean only, braised 1 raw chop with refuse, (113 g)	149	60	21	0	7	54	31	0.0
Pork, fresh, loin, top loin (chops), boneless, separable lean only, broiled 1 raw chop with refuse, (113 g)	134	48	20	0	5	53	43	0.0
Pork, fresh, loin, top loin (chops), boneless, separable lean only, pan-fried 1 raw chop with refuse, (113 g)	142	57	19	0	6	49	36	0.0
Pork, fresh, loin, top loin (roasts), boneless, separable lean and fat, roasted 3 oz (85g)	192	84	25	0	9	66	37	0.0
Pork, fresh, loin, top loin (roasts), boneless, separable lean only, roasted 3 oz (85g)	165	54	26	0	6	66	38	0.0
Pork, fresh, loin, whole, separable lean and fat, braised 3 oz (85g)	203	107	23	0	12	68	41	0.0
Pork, fresh, loin, whole, separable lean and fat, broiled 3 oz (85g)	206	107	23	0	12	68	53	0.0
Pork, fresh, loin, whole, separable lean and fat, roasted 3 oz (85g)	211	115	23	0	13	70	50	0.0
Pork, fresh, loin, whole, separable lean only, braised 1 raw chop with refuse, (151 g)	163	65	23	0	7	63	40	0.0
Pork, fresh, loin, whole, separable lean only, broiled 1 raw chop with refuse, (151 g)	166	71	23	0	8	62	51	0.0
Pork, fresh, loin, whole, separable lean only, roasted 1 raw chop with refuse, (151 g)	169	73	23	0	8	66	47	0.0
Pork, fresh, shoulder, arm picnic, separable lean and fat, braised 3 oz (85g)	280	176	24	0	20	93	75	0.0
Pork, fresh, shoulder, arm picnic, separable lean and fat, roasted 3 oz (85g)	269	184	20	0	20	80	60	0.0

Food Serving size	Cal.	Fat cal.	Prot.	Carb.	Fat	Chol.	Sod.	Fiber
Pork, fresh, shoulder, arm picnic, separable lean only, braised								
3 oz (85g)	211	92	27	0	10	97	87	0.0
Pork, fresh, shoulder, arm picnic, separable lean only, roasted								
3 oz (85g)	194	100	23	0	11	81	68	0.0
Pork, fresh, shoulder, blade, boston (roasts), separable lean and fat, roasted								
3 oz (85g)	229	146	20	0	16	73	57	0.0
Pork, fresh, shoulder, blade, boston (roasts), separable lean only, roasted								
3 oz (85g)	197	107	20	0	12	72	75	0.0
Pork, fresh, shoulder, blade, boston (steaks), separable lean and fat, braised								
3 oz (85g)	271	169	25	0	19	96	60	0.0
Pork, fresh, shoulder, blade, boston (steaks), separable lean and fat, broiled								
3 oz (85g)	220	130	22	0	14	81	59	0.0
Pork, fresh, shoulder, blade, boston (steaks), separable lean only, braised								
3 oz (85g)	232	123	26	0	14	99	64	0.0
Pork, fresh, shoulder, blade, boston (steaks), separable lean only, broiled								
3 oz (85g)	193	100	23	0	11	80	63	0.0
Pork, fresh, shoulder, whole, separable lean and fat, roasted								
3 oz (85g)	248	161	20	0	18	77	58	0.0
Pork, fresh, shoulder, whole, separable lean only, roasted								
3 oz (85g)	196	107	21	0	12	77	64	0.0
Pork, fresh, spareribs, separable lean and fat, braised								
3 oz (85g)	337	230	25	0	26	103	79	0.0
Pork, fresh, variety meats and by-products, brain, braised								
3 oz (85g)	117	77	10	0	9	2169	77	0.0
Pork, fresh, variety meats and by-products, chitterlings, simmered								
3 oz (85g)	258	222	9	0	25	122	33	0.0
Pork, fresh, variety meats and by-products, feet, simmered								
3 oz (85g)	165	92	16	0	10	85	26	0.0

Food Serving size	Cal.	Fat cal.	Prot.	Carb.	Fat	Chol.	Sod.	Fiber
Pork, fresh, variety meats and by-products, tongue, braised								
3 oz (85g)	230	146	20	0	16	124	93	0.0

Cured Pork

	Cal.	Fat cal.	Prot.	Carb.	Fat	Chol.	Sod.	Fiber
Pork, cured, Canadian-style bacon, grilled 2 slices (6 per 6-oz pkg.) (46g)	85	33	11	0	4	27	711	0.0
Pork, cured, Canadian-style bacon, unheated 2 slices (6 per 6-oz pkg.) (57g)	89	36	12	1	4	29	803	0.0
Pork, cured, bacon, broiled, pan-fried or roasted 3 medium slices packed 20/lb raw, after cooking	109	84	6	0	9	16	303	0.0
Pork, cured, breakfast strips, cooked 3 slices packed 15/12-oz bag, after cooking	156	113	10	0	13	36	714	0.0
Pork, cured, ham, boneless, extra lean (approximately 5% fat), roasted 3 oz (85g)	123	46	18	2	5	45	1023	0.0
Pork, cured, ham, boneless, extra lean and regular, roasted 3 oz (85g)	140	61	19	0	7	48	1177	0.0
Pork, cured, ham, boneless, extra lean and regular, unheated 1 slice $(6\frac{1}{4}'' \times 4'' \times \frac{1}{16}'')$ (1 oz)	45	20	5	1	2	15	358	0.0
Pork, cured, ham, boneless, regular (approximately 11% fat), roasted 3 oz (85g)	151	69	20	0	8	50	1275	0.0
Pork, cured, ham, center slice, separable lean and fat, unheated 1 oz (28g)	57	33	6	0	4	15	388	0.0
Pork, cured, ham, extra lean (approximately 4% fat), canned, roasted 3 oz (85g)	116	38	18	1	4	26	965	0.0
Pork, cured, ham, extra lean (approximately 4% fat), canned, unheated 1 oz (28g)	34	13	5	0	1	11	351	0.0

Food Serving size	Cal.	Fat cal.	Prot.	Carb.	Fat	Chol.	Sod.	Fiber
Pork, cured, ham, extra lean and regular, canned, roasted								
3 oz (85g)	142	61	18	0	7	35	908	0.0
Pork, cured, ham, extra lean and regular, canned, unheated								
1 oz (28g)	40	18	5	0	2	11	357	0.0
Pork, cured, ham, patties, grilled								
1 patty, cooked (60g)	205	168	8	1	19	43	638	0.0
Pork, cured, ham, regular (approximately 13% fat), canned, roasted								
3 oz (85g)	192	115	18	0	13	53	800	0.0
Pork, cured, ham, regular (approximately 13% fat), canned, unheated								
1 oz (28g)	53	33	5	0	4	11	347	0.0
Pork, cured, ham, steak, boneless, extra lean, unheated								
1 oz (28g)	34	10	6	0	1	13	355	0.0
Pork, cured, ham, whole, separable lean and fat, roasted								
3 oz (85g)	207	130	19	0	14	53	1009	0.0
Pork, cured, ham, whole, separable lean and fat, unheated								
1 oz (28g)	69	48	5	0	5	16	360	0.0
Pork, cured, ham, whole, separable lean only, roasted								
3 oz (85g)	133	46	21	0	5	47	1128	0.0
Pork, cured, ham, whole, separable lean only, unheated								
1 oz (28g)	41	15	6	0	2	15	424	0.0
Pork, cured, separable fat (from ham and arm picnic), roasted								
1 oz (28g)	165	157	2	0	17	24	175	0.0
Pork, cured, separable fat (from ham and arm picnic), unheated								
1 oz (28g)	162	154	2	0	17	19	141	0.0
Pork, cured, shoulder, arm picnic, separable lean and fat, roasted								
3 oz (85g)	238	161	17	0	18	49	911	0.0
Pork, cured, shoulder, arm picnic, separable lean only, roasted								
3 oz (85g)	145	54	21	0	6	41	1046	0.0
Pork, cured, shoulder, blade roll, separable lean and fat, roasted								
3 oz (85g)	244	176	14	0	20	57	827	0.0
Pork, cured, shoulder, blade roll, separable lean and fat, unheated								
1 oz (28g)	75	56	4	0	6	15	350	0.0

Poultry Products

Food Serving size	Cal.	Fat cal.	Prot.	Carb.	Fat	Chol.	Sod.	Fiber

Chicken

Chicken, broilers or fryers, back, meat and skin, fried, batter
From 1 lb ready to
cook chicken (72g) | 238 | 143 | 16 | 7 | 16 | 63 | 228 |

Chicken, broilers or fryers, back, meat and skin, fried, flour
From 1 lb ready to
cook chicken (44g) | 146 | 83 | 12 | 3 | 9 | 39 | 40 |

Chicken, broilers or fryers, back, meat and skin, roasted
From 1 lb ready to
cook chicken (32g) | 96 | 61 | 8 | 0 | 7 | 28 | 28 | 0.0 |

Chicken, broilers or fryers, back, meat and skin, stewed
From 1 lb ready to
cook chicken (36g) | 93 | 58 | 8 | 0 | 6 | 28 | 23 | 0.0 |

Chicken, broilers or fryers, back, meat only, fried
From 1 lb ready to
cook chicken (35g) | 101 | 47 | 11 | 2 | 5 | 33 | 35 | 0.0 |

Chicken, broilers or fryers, back, meat only, roasted
From 1 lb ready to
cook chicken (24g) | 57 | 28 | 7 | 0 | 3 | 22 | 23 | 0.0 |

Chicken, broilers or fryers, back, meat only, stewed
From 1 lb ready to
cook chicken (26g) | 54 | 26 | 7 | 0 | 3 | 22 | 17 | 0.0 |

Chicken, broilers or fryers, breast, meat and skin, fried, batter
From 1 lb ready to
cook chicken (84g) | 218 | 98 | 21 | 8 | 11 | 71 | 231 | 0.0 |

Food
Serving size   Cal. Fat cal. Prot. Carb. Fat Chol. Sod. Fiber

Food / Serving size	Cal.	Fat cal.	Prot.	Carb.	Fat	Chol.	Sod.	Fiber
Chicken, broilers or fryers, breast, meat and skin, fried, flour From 1 lb ready to cook chicken (59g)	131	48	19	1	5	53	45	0.0
Chicken, broilers or fryers, breast, meat and skin, roasted From 1 lb ready to cook chicken (58g)	114	42	17	0	5	49	41	0.0
Chicken, broilers or fryers, breast, meat and skin, stewed From 1 lb ready to cook chicken (66g)	121	42	18	0	5	50	41	0.0
Chicken, broilers or fryers, breast, meat only, fried From 1 lb ready to cook chicken (52g)	97	23	17	1	3	47	41	0.0
Chicken, broilers or fryers, breast, meat only, roasted From 1 lb ready to cook chicken (52g)	86	19	16	0	2	44	38	0.0
Chicken, broilers or fryers, breast, meat only, stewed From 1 lb ready to cook chicken (57g)	86	15	17	0	2	44	36	0.0
Chicken, broilers or fryers, dark meat, meat and skin, fried, batter From 1 lb ready to cook chicken (167g)	498	286	37	15	32	149	493	
Chicken, broilers or fryers, dark meat, meat and skin, fried, flour From 1 lb ready to cook chicken (110g)	314	169	30	4	19	101	98	
Chicken, broilers or fryers, dark meat, meat and skin, roasted From 1 lb ready to cook chicken (101g)	256	146	26	0	16	92	88	0.0
Chicken, broilers or fryers, dark meat, meat and skin, stewed From 1 lb ready to cook chicken (110g)	256	149	26	0	17	90	77	0.0
Chicken, broilers or fryers, dark meat, meat only, fried From 1 lb ready to cook chicken (91g)	217	98	26	3	11	87	88	0.0
Chicken, broilers or fryers, dark meat, meat only, roasted From 1 lb ready to cook chicken (81g)	166	73	22	0	8	75	75	0.0
Chicken, broilers or fryers, dark meat, meat only, stewed From 1 lb ready to cook chicken (86g)	165	70	22	0	8	76	64	0.0

Food Serving size	Cal.	Fat cal.	Prot.	Carb.	Fat	Chol.	Sod.	Fiber
Chicken, broilers or fryers, drumstick, meat and skin, fried, batter From 1 lb ready to cook chicken (43g)	115	62	9	3	7	37	116	0.0
Chicken, broilers or fryers, drumstick, meat and skin, fried, flour From 1 lb ready to cook chicken (29g)	71	37	8	1	4	26	26	0.0
Chicken, broilers or fryers, drumstick, meat and skin, roasted From 1 lb ready to cook chicken (31g)	67	31	8	0	3	28	28	0.0
Chicken, broilers or fryers, drumstick, meat and skin, stewed From 1 lb ready to cook chicken (34g)	69	34	9	0	4	28	26	0.0
Chicken, broilers or fryers, drumstick, meat only, fried From 1 lb ready to cook chicken (25g)	49	18	7	0	2	24	24	0.0
Chicken, broilers or fryers, drumstick, meat only, roasted From 1 lb ready to cook chicken (26g)	45	14	7	0	2	24	25	0.0
Chicken, broilers or fryers, drumstick, meat only, stewed From 1 lb ready to cook chicken (28g)	47	15	8	0	2	25	22	0.0
Chicken, broilers or fryers, giblets, fried From 1 lb ready to cook chicken (13g)	36	15	4	1	2	58	15	0.0
Chicken, broilers or fryers, giblets, simmered From 1 lb ready to cook chicken (14g)	22	6	4	0	1	55	8	0.0
Chicken, broilers or fryers, leg, meat and skin, fried, batter From 1 lb ready to cook chicken (95g)	259	137	21	9	15	86	265	0.0
Chicken, broilers or fryers, leg, meat and skin, fried, flour From 1 lb ready to cook chicken (67g)	170	85	18	1	9	63	59	0.0
Chicken, broilers or fryers, leg, meat and skin, roasted From 1 lb ready to cook chicken (69g)	160	81	18	0	9	63	60	0.0
Chicken, broilers or fryers, leg, meat and skin, stewed From 1 lb ready to cook chicken (75g)	165	88	18	0	10	63	55	0.0

Food Serving size	Cal.	Fat cal.	Prot.	Carb.	Fat	Chol.	Sod.	Fiber
Chicken, broilers or fryers, leg, meat only, fried From 1 lb ready to cook chicken (56g)	116	45	16	1	5	55	54	0.0
Chicken, broilers or fryers, leg, meat only, roasted From 1 lb ready to cook chicken (57g)	109	41	15	0	5	54	52	0.0
Chicken, broilers or fryers, leg, meat only, stewed From 1 lb ready to cook chicken (60g)	111	43	16	0	5	53	47	0.0
Chicken, broilers or fryers, light meat, meat and skin, fried, batter From 1 lb ready to cook chicken (113g)	313	153	27	11	17	95	324	
Chicken, broilers or fryers, light meat, meat and skin, fried, flour From 1 lb ready to cook chicken (78g)	192	84	23	2	9	68	60	0.0
Chicken, broilers or fryers, light meat, meat and skin, roasted From 1 lb ready to cook chicken (79g)	175	78	23	0	9	66	59	0.0
Chicken, broilers or fryers, light meat, meat and skin, stewed From 1 lb ready to cook chicken (90g)	181	81	23	0	9	67	57	0.0
Chicken, broilers or fryers, light meat, meat only, fried From 1 lb ready to cook chicken (64g)	123	35	21	0	4	58	52	0.0
Chicken, broilers or fryers, light meat, meat only, roasted From 1 lb ready to cook chicken (64g)	111	29	20	0	3	54	49	0.0
Chicken, broilers or fryers, light meat, meat only, stewed From 1 lb ready to cook chicken (71g)	113	26	21	0	3	55	46	0.0
Chicken, broilers or fryers, meat and skin, roasted 1 cup, chopped or diced (140g)	335	177	38	0	20	123	115	0.0
Chicken, broilers or fryers, meat and skin, stewed 1 cup, chopped or diced (140g)	307	164	35	0	18	109	94	0.0
Chicken, broilers or fryers, meat only, fried 1 cup, chopped or diced (140g)	307	114	43	3	13	132	127	0.0

Food Serving size	Cal.	Fat cal.	Prot.	Carb.	Fat	Chol.	Sod.	Fiber
Chicken, broilers or fryers, meat only, roasted 1 tablespoon (9g)	17	6	3	0	1	8	8	0.0
Chicken, broilers or fryers, meat only, stewed 1 tablespoon (9g)	16	6	2	0	1	7	6	0.0
Chicken, broilers or fryers, thigh, meat and skin, fried, batter From 1 lb ready to cook chicken (52g)	144	80	11	5	9	48	150	0.0
Chicken, broilers or fryers, thigh, meat and skin, fried, flour From 1 lb ready to cook chicken (38g)	100	51	10	1	6	37	33	0.0
Chicken, broilers or fryers, thigh, meat and skin, roasted From 1 lb ready to cook chicken (37g)	91	50	9	0	6	34	31	0.0
Chicken, broilers or fryers, thigh, meat and skin, stewed From 1 lb ready to cook chicken (41g)	95	55	9	0	6	34	29	0.0
Chicken, broilers or fryers, thigh, meat only, fried From 1 lb ready to cook chicken (31g)	68	28	9	0	3	32	29	0.0
Chicken, broilers or fryers, thigh, meat only, roasted From 1 lb ready to cook chicken (31g)	65	31	8	0	3	29	27	0.0
Chicken, broilers or fryers, thigh, meat only, stewed From 1 lb ready to cook chicken (33g)	64	30	8	0	3	30	25	0.0
Chicken, broilers or fryers, wing, meat and skin, fried, batter From 1 lb ready to cook chicken (29g)	94	58	6	3	6	23	93	0.0
Chicken, broilers or fryers, wing, meat and skin, fried, flour From 1 lb ready to cook chicken (19g)	61	38	5	0	4	15	15	0.0
Chicken, broilers or fryers, wing, meat and skin, roasted From 1 lb ready to cook chicken (21g)	61	36	6	0	4	18	17	0.0
Chicken, broilers or fryers, wing, meat and skin, stewed From 1 lb ready to cook chicken (24g)	60	37	6	0	4	17	16	0.0

Food Serving size	Cal.	Fat cal.	Prot.	Carb.	Fat	Chol.	Sod.	Fiber
Chicken, broilers or fryers, wing, meat only, fried From 1 lb ready to cook chicken (12g)	25	10	4	0	1	10	11	0.0
Chicken, broilers or fryers, wing, meat only, roasted From 1 lb ready to cook chicken (13g)	26	9	4	0	1	11	12	0.0
Chicken, broilers or fryers, wing, meat only, stewed From 1 lb ready to cook chicken (14g)	25	9	4	0	1	10	10	0.0
Chicken, canned, meat only, with broth 1 can (5 oz) (142g)	234	102	31	0	11	88	714	0.0
Chicken, capons, meat and skin, roasted From 1 lb ready-to-cook capon (196g)	449	212	57	0	24	169	96	0.0
Chicken, cornish game hens, meat and skin, roasted ½ bird (129g)	335	209	28	0	23	169	83	0.0
Chicken, cornish game hens, meat only, roasted ½ bird (110g)	147	40	25	0	4	117	69	0.0
Chicken, liver, all classes, simmered From 1 lb ready to cook chicken (6g)	9	3	1	0	0	38	3	0.0

Turkey

Food Serving size	Cal.	Fat cal.	Prot.	Carb.	Fat	Chol.	Sod.	Fiber
Turkey, all classes, back, meat and skin, roasted 1 cup, chopped or diced (140g)	340	177	38	0	20	127	102	0.0
Turkey, all classes, breast, meat and skin, roasted From 1 lb ready to cook turkey (112g)	212	71	32	0	8	83	71	0.0
Turkey, all classes, dark meat, roasted From 1 lb ready to cook turkey (91g)	170	57	26	0	6	77	72	0.0
Turkey, all classes, dark meat, meat and skin, roasted From 1 lb ready to cook turkey (104g)	230	113	28	0	12	93	79	0.0

Food Serving size	Cal.	Fat cal.	Prot.	Carb.	Fat	Chol.	Sod.	Fiber
Turkey, all classes, giblets, simmered, some giblet fat From 1 lb ready to cook turkey (10g)	17	5	3	0	1	42	6	0.0
Turkey, all classes, leg, meat and skin, roasted From 1 lb ready to cook turkey (71g)	148	64	20	0	7	60	55	0.0
Turkey, all classes, light meat, roasted From 1 lb ready to cook turkey (117g)	184	32	35	0	4	81	75	0.0
Turkey, all classes, light meat, meat and skin, roasted From 1 lb ready to cook turkey (136g)	268	98	39	0	11	103	86	0.0
Turkey, all classes, meat and skin, roasted 1 cup, chopped or diced (140g)	291	126	39	0	14	115	95	0.0
Turkey, all classes, meat only, roasted 1 cup, chopped or diced (140g)	238	63	41	0	7	106	98	0.0
Turkey, all classes, wing, meat and skin, roasted From 1 lb ready to cook turkey (24g)	55	26	6	0	3	19	15	0.0
Turkey, canned, meat only, with broth 1 cup, drained (135g)	220	85	32	0	9	89	630	0.0
Turkey, diced, light and dark meat, seasoned 1 oz (28g)	39	15	5	0	2	15	238	0.0
Turkey, fryer-roasters, back, meat and skin, roasted From 1 lb ready to cook turkey (37g)	75	33	10	0	4	40	26	0.0
Turkey, fryer-roasters, back, meat only, roasted From 1 lb ready to cook turkey (27g)	46	15	8	0	2	26	20	0.0
Turkey, fryer-roasters, breast, meat and skin, roasted From 1 lb ready to cook turkey (98g)	150	27	28	0	3	88	52	0.0
Turkey, fryer-roasters, breast, meat only, roasted From 1 lb ready to cook turkey (87g)	117	8	26	0	1	72	45	0.0

Food Serving size	Cal.	Fat cal.	Prot.	Carb.	Fat	Chol.	Sod.	Fiber
Turkey, fryer-roasters, dark meat, meat and skin, roasted From 1 lb ready to cook turkey (106g)	193	67	30	0	7	124	81	0.0
Turkey, fryer-roasters, dark meat, meat only, roasted From 1 lb ready to cook turkey (91g)	147	33	26	0	4	102	72	0.0
Turkey, fryer-roasters, leg, meat and skin, roasted From 1 lb ready to cook turkey (70g)	119	32	20	0	4	49	56	0.0
Turkey, fryer-roasters, leg, meat only, roasted From 1 lb ready to cook turkey (64g)	102	23	19	0	3	76	52	0.0
Turkey, fryer-roasters, light meat, meat and skin, roasted From 1 lb ready to cook turkey (123g)	202	55	36	0	6	117	70	0.0
Turkey, fryer-roasters, light meat, meat only, roasted From 1 lb ready to cook turkey (104g)	146	9	31	0	1	89	58	0.0
Turkey, fryer-roasters, meat and skin and giblets and neck, roasted From 1 lb ready to cook turkey (251g)	429	136	70	0	15	296	163	0.0
Turkey, fryer-roasters, meat and skin, roasted From 1 lb ready to cook turkey (229g)	394	124	64	0	14	240	151	0.0
Turkey, fryer-roasters, meat only, roasted 1 cup, chopped or diced (140g)	210	38	42	0	4	137	94	0.0
Turkey, fryer-roasters, wing, meat and skin, roasted From 1 lb ready to cook turkey (25g)	52	23	7	0	3	29	18	0.0
Turkey, fryer-roasters, wing, meat only, roasted From 1 lb ready to cook turkey (17g)	28	5	5	0	1	17	13	0.0
Turkey, gizzard, all classes, simmered From 1 lb ready to cook turkey (4g)	7	1	1	0	0	9	2	0.0
Turkey, young hen, back, meat and skin, roasted From 1 lb ready to cook turkey (35g)	89	51	9	0	6	30	24	0.0

Food Serving size	Cal.	Fat cal.	Prot.	Carb.	Fat	Chol.	Sod.	Fiber
Turkey, young hen, breast, meat and skin, roasted From 1 lb ready to cook turkey (109g)	211	79	32	0	9	78	63	0.0
Turkey, young hen, dark meat, meat and skin, roasted From 1 lb ready to cook turkey (106g)	246	124	29	0	14	89	76	0.0
Turkey, young hen, dark meat, meat only, roasted From 1 lb ready to cook turkey (93g)	179	67	26	0	7	74	70	0.0
Turkey, young hen, leg, meat and skin, roasted From 1 lb ready to cook turkey (71g)	151	64	20	0	7	58	52	0.0
Turkey, young hen, light meat, meat and skin, roasted From 1 lb ready to cook turkey (137g)	284	111	40	0	12	101	79	0.0
Turkey, young hen, light meat, meat only, roasted From 1 lb ready to cook turkey (119g)	192	43	36	0	5	81	71	0.0
Turkey, young hen, meat and skin, roasted From 1 lb ready to cook turkey (243g)	530	241	68	0	27	190	156	0.0
Turkey, young hen, meat only, roasted 1 cup, chopped or diced (140g)	245	76	41	0	8	102	94	0.0
Turkey, young hen, wing, meat and skin, roasted From 1 lb ready to cook turkey (28g)	67	33	8	0	4	22	16	0.0
Turkey, young tom, back, meat and skin, roasted From 1 lb ready to cook turkey (33g)	79	42	9	0	5	31	25	0.0
Turkey, young tom, breast, meat and skin, roasted From 1 lb ready to cook turkey (115g)	217	73	33	0	8	86	77	0.0
Turkey, young tom, dark meat, meat and skin, roasted From 1 lb ready to cook turkey (103g)	222	102	29	0	11	94	82	0.0
Turkey, young tom, dark meat, meat only, roasted From 1 lb ready to cook turkey (90g)	167	57	26	0	6	79	74	0.0

Food Serving size	Cal.	Fat cal.	Prot.	Carb.	Fat	Chol.	Sod.	Fiber
Turkey, young tom, leg, meat and skin, roasted From 1 lb ready to cook turkey (70g)	144	63	20	0	7	63	56	0.0
Turkey, young tom, light meat, meat and skin, roasted From 1 lb ready to cook turkey (136g)	260	98	38	0	11	102	91	0.0
Turkey, young tom, light meat, meat only, roasted From 1 lb ready to cook turkey (117g)	180	32	35	0	4	81	80	0.0
Turkey, young tom, meat and skin, roasted From 1 lb ready to cook turkey (239g)	483	194	67	0	22	196	172	0.0
Turkey, young tom, meat only, roasted 1 cup, chopped or diced (140g)	235	63	41	0	7	108	104	0.0
Turkey, young tom, wing, meat and skin, roasted From 1 lb ready to cook turkey (21g)	46	23	6	0	3	17	14	0.0
Turkey and gravy, frozen 1 package, (net weight, 5 oz) (142g)	95	38	9	7	4	26	787	0.0
Turkey breast, pre-basted, meat and skin, roasted $\frac{1}{2}$ breast, bone removed (864g)	1089	234	190	0	26	363	3430	0.0
Turkey patties, breaded, battered, fried 1 medium slice (approx 3″ x 2″ x $\frac{1}{4}$″)	79	45	4	4	5	17	224	0.0
Turkey roast, boneless, frozen, seasoned, light and dark meat, roasted 1 cup, chopped or diced (135g)	209	73	28	4	8	72	918	0.0
Turkey sticks, breaded, battered, fried 1 stick (2.25 oz) (64g)	179	98	9	11	11	41	536	
Turkey thigh, pre-basted, meat and skin, roasted 1 thigh, bone removed (314g)	493	255	60	0	28	195	1372	0.0

Food Serving size	Cal.	Fat cal.	Prot.	Carb.	Fat	Chol.	Sod.	Fiber

Miscellaneous Poultry

Duck, domesticated, meat and skin, roasted
1 cup, chopped or diced

(140g)	472	354	27	0	39	118	83	0.0

Duck, domesticated, meat only, roasted
From 1 lb ready to

cook duck (100g)	201	99	23	0	11	89	65	0.0

Duck, young duckling, domesticated, White Pekin, breast, meat and skin, boneless, roasted
From 1 lb ready to

cook duck (56g)	113	56	13	0	6	76	47	

Duck, young duckling, domesticated, White Pekin, breast, meat only, boneless, cooked without skin, broiled
From 1 lb ready to

cook duck (44g)	62	8	12	0	1	63	46	

Duck, young duckling, domesticated, White Pekin, leg, meat and skin, bone in, roasted
From 1 lb ready to

cook duck (43g)	93	43	12	0	5	49	47	

Duck, young duckling, domesticated, White Pekin, leg, meat only, bone in, cooked without skin, braised
From 1 lb ready to

cook duck (35g)	62	19	10	0	2	37	38	

Goose, domesticated, meat and skin, roasted
1 cup, chopped or diced

(140g)	427	278	35	0	31	127	98	0.0

Goose, domesticated, meat only, roasted
From 1 lb ready to

cook goose (143g)	340	168	41	0	19	137	109	0.0

Pâté de foie gras, canned (goose liver pate), smoked

1 tablespoon (13g)	60	52	1	1	6	20	91	0.0

Baked Products

Food Serving size	Cal.	Fat cal.	Prot.	Carb.	Fat	Chol.	Sod.	Fiber

Breads

Bagels, cinnamon-raisin, toasted

1 oz (28g)	82	0	3	17	1	0	97	0.6

Bagels, cinnamon-raisin

1 oz (28g)	77	5	3	15	1	0	90	0.6

Bagels, egg, toasted

1 oz (28g)	84	0	3	16	1	7	152	0.6

Bagels, egg

1 oz (28g)	78	5	3	15	1	7	141	0.6

Bagels, oat bran, toasted

1 oz (28g)	77	0	3	16	0	0	153	1.1

Bagels, oat bran

1 oz (28g)	71	2	3	15	0	0	142	1.1

Bagels, plain, enriched, with calcium propionate (includes onion, poppy, sesame)

1 oz (28g)	77	5	3	15	1	0	150	0.6

Bagels, plain, enriched, without calcium propionate (includes onion, poppy, sesame)

1 oz (28g)	77	5	3	15	1	0	150	0.6

Bagels, plain, toasted, enriched, with calcium propionate (includes onion, poppy, sesame)

1 oz (28g)	83	0	3	16	1	0	161	0.6

Bagels, plain, toasted, enriched, without calcium propionate (includes onion, poppy, sesame)

1 oz (28g)	83	0	3	16	1	0	161	0.6

Food Serving size	Cal.	Fat cal.	Prot.	Carb.	Fat	Chol.	Sod.	Fiber
Bagels, plain, toasted, unenriched, with calcium propionate (includes onion, poppy, sesame)								
1 oz (28g)	83	0	3	16	1	0	161	
Bagels, plain, toasted, unenriched, without calcium propionate (includes onion, poppy, sesame)								
1 oz (28g)	83		3	16	1	0	161	
Bagels, plain, unenriched, with calcium propionate (includes onion, poppy, sesame)								
1 oz (28g)	77	5	3	15	1	0	150	0.6
Bagels, plain, unenriched, without calcium propionate (includes onion, poppy, sesame)								
1 oz (28g)	77	5	3	15	1	0	150	0.6
Biscuits, mixed grain, refrigerated dough, baked								
1 oz (28g)	85	0	2	15	2	0	218	0.8
Biscuits, plain or buttermilk, commercially baked								
1 oz (28g)	102	39	2	13	4	0	295	0.3
Biscuits, plain or buttermilk, dry mix, prepared								
1 oz (28g)	94	0	2	13	3	1	267	0.6
Biscuits, plain or buttermilk, prepared from recipe								
1 oz (28g)	99	0	2	13	4	1	162	0.6
Biscuits, plain or buttermilk, refrigerated dough, higher fat, baked 1 biscuit ($2\frac{1}{2}''$ dia)								
(27g)	93	0	2	13	4	0	325	0.5
Biscuits, plain or buttermilk, refrigerated dough, lower fat, baked 1 biscuit ($2\frac{1}{4}''$ dia)								
(21g)	63	0	2	12	1	0	305	0.4
Bread crumbs, dry, grated, plain								
1 oz (28g)	111	12	3	20	1	0	241	0.6
Bread crumbs, dry, grated, seasoned								
1 oz (28g)	103	7	4	20	1	1	742	1.1
Bread sticks, plain 1 small stick (approx $4\frac{1}{4}''$ long) (5g)	21	4	1	3	1	0	33	0.2
Bread stuffing, bread, dry mix, prepared								
1 oz (28g)	50	0	1	6	3	0	152	0.8

Food Serving size	Cal.	Fat cal.	Prot.	Carb.	Fat	Chol.	Sod.	Fiber
Bread stuffing, cornbread, dry mix, prepared								
1 oz (28g)	50	0	1	6	3	0	127	0.8
Bread stuffing, plain, prepared from recipe								
1 oz (28g)	47	0	1	6	2	0	129	
Bread, banana, prepared from recipe, made with margarine								
1 oz (28g)	91	0	1	15	3	12	85	0.3
Bread, banana, prepared from recipe, made with vegetable shortening								
1 oz (28g)	95	0	1	15	3	12	55	
Bread, Boston brown, canned								
1 oz (28g)	55	5	1	12	1	0	177	1.4
Bread, cornbread, dry mix, enriched (includes corn muffin mix)								
1 oz (28g)	117	30	2	20	3	0	311	1.7
Bread, cornbread, dry mix, prepared								
1 oz (28g)	88	0	2	13	3	17	218	0.6
Bread, cornbread, dry mix, unenriched (includes corn muffin mix)								
1 oz (28g)	117	28	2	20	3	0	311	1.7
Bread, cornbread, prepared from recipe, made with low fat (2%) milk								
1 oz (28g)	74	0	2	12	2	11	184	
Bread, cornbread, prepared from recipe, made with whole milk								
1 oz (28g)	76	0	2	12	2	12	184	1.1
Bread, cracked-wheat, toasted 1 large or thick slice								
(27g)	76	0	3	15	1	0	158	1.6
Bread, cracked-wheat								
1 cubic inch (3g)	8	1	0	2	0	0	16	0.2
Bread, egg, toasted								
1 oz (28g)	88	0	3	15	2	16	151	0.6
Bread, egg								
1 oz (28g)	80	0	3	13	2	14	138	0.6
Bread, French or Vienna (includes sourdough)								
1 oz (28g)	77	7	3	15	1	0	171	0.8
Bread, French or Vienna, toasted (includes sourdough)								
1 oz (28g)	83	0	3	16	1	0	185	0.8

Food Serving size	Cal.	Fat cal.	Prot.	Carb.	Fat	Chol.	Sod.	Fiber
Bread, Indian (Navajo) fry 5″ diameter (90g)	296	0	6	48	9	0	626	1.8
Bread, Irish soda, prepared from recipe 1 oz (28g)	81	0	2	16	1	5	111	0.8
Bread, Italian, toasted 1 large slice ($4\frac{1}{2}''$ x $3\frac{1}{4}''$ x $\frac{3}{4}''$)	80	0	3	15	1	0	173	0.8
Bread, Italian 1 oz (28g)	76	10	3	14	1	0	164	0.8
Bread, mixed-grain (includes whole-grain, 7-grain) 1 oz (28g)	70	10	3	13	1	0	136	1.7
Bread, mixed-grain, toasted (includes whole-grain, 7-grain) 1 oz (28g)	76	0	3	14	1	0	148	2.0
Bread, oat bran, toasted 1 slice (27g)	70	0	3	12	1	0	121	1.4
Bread, oat bran 1 oz (28g)	66	10	3	11	1	0	114	1.1
Bread, oatmeal, toasted 1 slice (25g)	73	0	2	13	1	0	163	1.0
Bread, oatmeal 1 slice (27g)	73	9	2	13	1	0	162	1.1
Bread, pita, white, enriched 1 small pita (4″ dia) (28g)	77	2	3	16	0	0	150	0.6
Bread, pita, white, unenriched 1 oz (28g)	77	2	3	16	0	0	150	0.6
Bread, pita, whole-wheat 1 small pita (4″ dia) (28g)	74	7	3	15	1	0	149	2.0
Bread, protein (includes gluten) 1 slice (19g)	47	3	2	8	0	0	104	0.6
Bread, protein, toasted (includes gluten) 1 slice (17g)	46	0	2	8	0	0	102	0.5
Bread, pumpernickel, toasted 1 oz (28g)	77	0	3	15	1	0	207	2.0

Food Serving size	Cal.	Fat cal.	Prot.	Carb.	Fat	Chol.	Sod.	Fiber
Bread, pumpernickel 1 regular slice (26g)	65	7	2	12	1	0	174	1.6
Bread, pumpkin, prepared from recipe 1 oz (28g)	93	0	1	14	4	12	88	
Bread, raisin, enriched 1 oz (28g)	77	10	2	15	1	0	109	1.1
Bread, raisin, toasted, enriched 1 oz (28g)	83	0	3	16	1	0	119	1.4
Bread, raisin, toasted, unenriched 1 oz (28g)	83	0	3	16	1	0	119	
Bread, raisin, unenriched 1 oz (28g)	77	10	2	15	1	0	109	
Bread, reduced-calorie, oat bran, toasted 1 slice (19g)	45	0	2	9	1	0	79	2.7
Bread, reduced-calorie, oat bran 1 slice (23g)	46	6	2	9	1	0	81	2.8
Bread, reduced-calorie, oatmeal, toasted 1 slice (19g)	48	0	2	10	1	0	88	
Bread, reduced-calorie, oatmeal 1 slice (23g)	48	8	2	10	1	0	89	
Bread, reduced-calorie, rye, toasted 1 slice (19g)	46	0	2	9	1	0	92	
Bread, reduced-calorie, rye 1 slice (23g)	47	6	2	9	1	0	93	2.8
Bread, reduced-calorie, wheat, toasted 1 slice (19g)	45	0	2	10	1	0	116	
Bread, reduced-calorie, wheat 1 slice (23g)	46	4	2	10	0	0	118	2.8
Bread, reduced-calorie, white, toasted 1 slice (19g)	47	0	2	10	1	0	102	
Bread, reduced-calorie, white 1 slice (23g)	48	4	2	10	0	0	104	2.3
Bread, rice bran, toasted 1 slice (25g)	66	0	3	12	1	0	120	1.3

Food Serving size	Cal.	Fat cal.	Prot.	Carb.	Fat	Chol.	Sod.	Fiber
Bread, rice bran 1 slice (27g)	66	12	2	12	1	0	119	1.4
Bread, rye, toasted 1 oz (28g)	80	0	3	15	1	0	203	1.7
Bread, rye 1 oz (28g)	73	7	2	13	1	0	185	1.7
Bread, wheat (includes wheat berry) 1 slice (25g)	65	9	2	12	1	0	133	1.0
Bread, wheat bran, toasted 1 oz (28g)	76	0	3	15	1	0	150	1.1
Bread, wheat bran 1 oz (28g)	69	7	3	13	1	0	136	1.1
Bread, wheat germ, toasted 1 slice (25g)	73	0	3	14	1	0	155	0.5
Bread, wheat germ 1 oz (28g)	73	7	3	13	1	0	155	0.6
Bread, wheat, toasted (includes wheat berry) 1 slice (23g)	65	0	2	12	1	0	132	1.1
Bread, white, commercially prepared (includes soft bread crumbs) 1 cup, cubes (35g)	93	12	3	18	1	0	188	0.7
Bread, white, commercially prepared, low sodium 1 cup, cubes (35g)	93	12	3	18	1	0	9	0.7
Bread, white, commercially prepared, toasted, low sodium 1 slice (23g)	67	8	2	12	1	0	7	
Bread, white, commercially prepared, toasted 1 cup, cubes (42g)	123	0	4	23	2	0	249	0.8
Bread, white, prepared from recipe, made with low fat (2%) milk, toasted 1 oz (28g)	88	0	3	15	2	1	110	0.6
Bread, white, prepared from recipe, made with low fat (2%) milk 1 oz (28g)	80	0	2	14	2	1	101	0.6
Bread, white, prepared from recipe, made with nonfat dry milk, toasted 1 oz (28g)	84	0	2	17	1	0	103	

Food Serving size	Cal.	Fat cal.	Prot.	Carb.	Fat	Chol.	Sod.	Fiber
Bread, white, prepared from recipe, made with nonfat dry milk								
1 oz (28g)	77	0	2	15	1	0	94	0.6
Bread, white, prepared from recipe, made with whole milk, toasted								
1 oz (28g)	89	0	3	15	2	2	110	
Bread, white, prepared from recipe, made with whole milk								
1 oz (28g)	81	0	2	14	2	1	101	
Bread, whole-wheat, commercially prepared, toasted								
1 slice (25g)	69	0	3	13	1	0	148	1.8
Bread, whole-wheat, commercially prepared								
1 oz (28g)	69	10	3	13	1	0	148	2.0
Bread, whole-wheat, prepared from recipe, toasted								
1 oz (28g)	85	0	3	16	2	0	107	2.0
Bread, whole-wheat, prepared from recipe								
1 oz (28g)	78	0	2	14	1	0	97	1.7

Cakes

Food Serving size	Cal.	Fat cal.	Prot.	Carb.	Fat	Chol.	Sod.	Fiber
Cake, angelfood, commercially prepared 1 piece ($\frac{1}{12}$ of 12 oz cake) (28g)	72	2	2	16	0	0	210	0.6
Cake, angelfood, dry mix, prepared 1 piece ($\frac{1}{12}$ of 10″ dia) (50g)	129	0	3	30	0	0	255	0.0
Cake, angelfood, prepared from recipe 1 oz (28g)	75	0	2	17	0	0	51	
Cake, Boston cream pie, commercially prepared 1 oz (28g)	71	20	1	12	2	10	40	0.3
Cake, Boston cream pie, prepared from recipe 1 oz (28g)	88	0	1	13	4	13	93	
Cake, carrot, dry mix, pudding-type, prepared without frosting 1 piece ($\frac{1}{12}$ of 9″ dia) (70g)	239	0	4	33	11	51	249	1.4
Cake, carrot, dry mix, pudding-type 1 oz (28g)	116	25	1	22	3	0	159	

Food Serving size	Cal.	Fat cal.	Prot.	Carb.	Fat	Chol.	Sod.	Fiber
Cake, carrot, prepared from recipe with cream cheese frosting								
1 oz (28g)	122	0	1	13	7	15	69	0.3
Cake, cherry fudge with chocolate frosting								
1 oz (28g)	74	30	1	11	3	15	63	0.3
Cake, chocolate, commercially prepared with chocolate frosting								
1 oz (28g)	103	39	1	15	4	13	94	0.8
Cake, chocolate, dry mix, pudding-type, prepared without frosting								
1 piece ($\frac{1}{12}$ of 9" dia)								
(77g)	270	0	4	34	15	53	402	1.5
Cake, chocolate, dry mix, regular, prepared without frosting								
1 piece ($\frac{1}{12}$ of 9" dia)								
(65g)	198	0	4	32	8	35	370	1.3
Cake, chocolate, dry mix, special dietary								
1 oz (28g)	108	24	1	22	3	0	115	
Cake, chocolate, prepared from recipe without frosting								
1 piece ($\frac{1}{12}$ of 9" dia)								
(95g)	340	0	5	50	14	55	299	1.9
Cake, fruitcake, commercially prepared								
1 oz (28g)	91	22	1	17	3	1	76	1.1
Cake, fruitcake, prepared from recipe								
1 oz (28g)	101	0	1	18	3	8	40	
Cake, German chocolate, dry mix, pudding-type, prepared with coconut-nut frosting								
1 oz (28g)	102	0	1	14	5	13	93	0.3
Cake, gingerbread, dry mix, prepared								
1 oz (28g)	87	0	1	14	3	10	128	0.3
Cake, gingerbread, prepared from recipe								
1 oz (28g)	100	0	1	14	4	9	92	
Cake, marble, dry mix, pudding-type, prepared without frosting								
1 piece ($\frac{1}{12}$ of 9" dia)								
(73g)	253	0	3	34	12	53	242	1.5
Cake, pineapple upside-down, prepared from recipe								
1 oz (28g)	89	0	1	14	3	6	89	0.3

Food Serving size	Cal.	Fat cal.	Prot.	Carb.	Fat	Chol.	Sod.	Fiber
Cake, pound, commercially prepared, butter 1 piece ($\frac{1}{12}$ of 12 oz cake) (28g)	109	49	2	14	6	62	111	0.0
Cake, pound, commercially prepared, fat-free 1 oz (28g)	79	2	1	17	0	0	95	0.3
Cake, pound, commercially prepared, other than all butter, enriched 1 piece ($\frac{1}{12}$ of 12 oz cake) (28g)	109	44	1	15	5	16	112	0.3
Cake, pound, commercially prepared, other than all butter, unenriched 1 piece ($\frac{1}{12}$ of 12 oz cake) (28g)	109	44	1	15	5	16	112	0.3
Cake, pound, prepared from recipe, modified, made with butter 1 oz (28g)	107	0	2	15	5	32	83	
Cake, pound, prepared from recipe, modified, made with margarine 1 oz (28g)	107	0	2	15	5	21	89	
Cake, pound, prepared from recipe, old-fashioned, made with butter 1 oz (28g)	121	0	2	13	7	48	81	
Cake, pound, prepared from recipe, old-fashioned, made with margarine 1 oz (28g)	122	0	2	13	7	32	89	
Cake, shortcake, biscuit-type, prepared from recipe 1 oz (28g)	97	0	2	13	4	1	142	
Cake, snack cakes, creme-filled, chocolate with frosting 1 oz (28g)	105	34	1	17	4	5	119	0.3
Cake, snack cakes, creme-filled, sponge 1 oz (28g)	102	27	1	18	3	4	102	0.0
Cake, snack cakes, cupcakes, chocolate, with frosting, low-fat 1 oz (28g)	85	10	1	19	1	0	116	1.1
Cake, sponge, commercially prepared 1 oz (28g)	81	0	1	17	1	29	68	0.3
Cake, sponge, prepared from recipe 1 oz (28g)	83	0	2	16	1	48	64	

Food Serving size	Cal.	Fat cal.	Prot.	Carb.	Fat	Chol.	Sod.	Fiber
Cake, white, dry mix, pudding-type, prepared without frosting 1 piece ($\frac{1}{12}$ of 9″ dia) (69g)	244	0	3	36	10	0	305	0.0
Cake, white, dry mix, regular, prepared without frosting 1 piece ($\frac{1}{12}$ of 9″ dia) (62g)	190	0	2	34	5	0	301	0.6
Cake, white, dry mix, special dietary, prepared without frosting 1 oz (28g)	87	0	1	17	2	0	61	0.3
Cake, white, prepared from recipe with coconut frosting 1 oz (28g)	100	0	1	18	3	0	80	0.3
Cake, white, prepared from recipe without frosting 1 piece ($\frac{1}{12}$ of 9″ dia) (74g)	264	0	4	42	9	1	242	0.7
Cake, yellow, commercially prepared, with chocolate frosting 1 oz (28g)	106	42	1	15	5	15	94	0.6
Cake, yellow, commercially prepared, with vanilla frosting 1 oz (28g)	104	35	1	17	4	16	96	0.0
Cake, yellow, dry mix, light, prepared without frosting, 3% fat 1 piece ($\frac{1}{12}$ of 9″ dia) (69g)	181	0	3	37	3	0	279	0.7
Cake, yellow, dry mix, pudding-type, prepared without frosting 1 piece ($\frac{1}{12}$ of 9″ dia) (73g)	257	0	3	35	12	53	317	0.0
Cake, yellow, dry mix, regular, prepared without frosting 1 piece ($\frac{1}{12}$ of 9″ dia) (63g)	202	0	3	34	6	37	299	0.6
Cake, yellow, prepared from recipe without frosting 1 piece ($\frac{1}{12}$ of 8″ dia) (68g)	245	0	3	36	10	37	233	0.7
Cheesecake commercially prepared 1 oz (28g)	90	54	2	7	6	15	58	0.0
Cheesecake prepared from mix, no-bake type 1 oz (28g)	77	32	2	10	4	12	106	0.6

Food Serving size	Cal.	Fat cal.	Prot.	Carb.	Fat	Chol.	Sod.	Fiber
Cheesecake prepared from recipe								
1 oz (28g)	100	0	2	7	7	34	79	
Cheesecake, plain, prepared from recipe, with cherry topping								
1 oz (28g)	80	0	1	7	5	24	57	
Coffeecake, cheese								
1 oz (28g)	95	37	2	12	4	10	95	0.3
Coffeecake, cinnamon with crumb topping, commercially prepared, enriched								
1 oz (28g)	117	57	2	13	6	9	98	0.6
Coffeecake, cinnamon with crumb topping, commercially prepared, unenriched								
1 oz (28g)	117	57	2	13	6	9	98	0.8
Coffeecake, cinnamon with crumb topping, dry mix, prepared								
1 oz (28g)	89	0	2	15	3	14	118	0.3
Coffeecake, cinnamon with crumb topping, prepared from recipe								
1 oz (28g)	112	0	2	14	6	17	109	
Coffeecake, creme-filled with chocolate frosting								
1 oz (28g)	93	27	1	15	3	7	90	0.6
Coffeecake, fruit								
1 oz (28g)	87	25	1	15	3	6	108	0.6

Cookies

Food Serving size	Cal.	Fat cal.	Prot.	Carb.	Fat	Chol.	Sod.	Fiber
Cookies, animal crackers (includes arrowroot, tea biscuits)								
1 Arrowroot biscuit	22	6	0	4	1	0	20	0.1
Cookies, brownies, commercially prepared								
1 oz (28g)	113	39	1	18	4	5	87	0.6
Cookies, brownies, dry mix, regular, prepared								
1 oz (28g)	118	0	1	17	6	8	71	0.8
Cookies, brownies, dry mix, special dietary, prepared 1 brownie (2″ square)								
(22g)	84	0	1	16	2	0	21	0.9
Cookies, brownies, prepared from recipe 1 brownie (2″ square)								
(24g)	112	0	1	12	7	18	82	

Food Serving size	Cal.	Fat cal.	Prot.	Carb.	Fat	Chol.	Sod.	Fiber
Cookies, butter, commercially prepared, enriched								
1 cookie (5g)	23	8	0	3	1	4	18	0.1
Cookies, butter, commercially prepared, unenriched								
1 cookie (5g)	23	8	0	3	1	4	18	0.1
Cookies, chocolate chip, commercially prepared, higher fat, unenriched 1 medium cookie								
$(2\frac{1}{4}''$ dia) (10g)	48	20	1	7	2	0	32	0.2
Cookies, chocolate chip, commercially prepared, reduced fat								
1 cookie (10g)	45	13	1	7	2	0	38	0.4
Cookies, chocolate chip, commercially prepared, soft-type								
1 cookie (15g)	69	32	1	9	4	0	49	0.4
Cookies, chocolate chip, commercially prepared, special dietary 1 medium cookie								
$(1\frac{5}{8}''$ dia) (7g)	32	10	0	5	1	0	1	0.1
Cookies, chocolate chip, dry mix, prepared								
1 cookie (2″ dia) (16g)	79	0	1	10	4	7	47	0.2
Cookies, chocolate chip, prepared from recipe, made with butter 1 medium cookie								
$(2\frac{1}{4}''$ dia) (16g)	78	0	1	9	4	11	55	
Cookies, chocolate chip, prepared from recipe, made with margarine								
1 oz (28g)	137	0	2	16	8	9	101	0.8
Cookies, chocolate chip, refrigerated dough, baked 1 medium cookie								
$(2\frac{1}{4}''$ dia) (12g)	59	0	1	8	3	3	28	0.2
Cookies, chocolate chip, refrigerated dough Dough for 1 cookie								
(16g)	71	28	1	10	3	4	33	0.2
Cookies, chocolate sandwich, with creme filling, chocolate-coated								
1 cookie (17g)	82	39	1	11	4	0	55	0.9
Cookies, chocolate sandwich, with creme filling								
1 cookie (10g)	47	18	1	7	2	0	60	0.3
Cookies, chocolate sandwich, with creme filling, special dietary								
1 cookie (10g)	46	19	0	7	2	0	24	0.4
Cookies, chocolate sandwich, with extra creme filling								
1 cookie (13g)	65	29	1	9	3	0	64	0.3

Food Serving size	Cal.	Fat cal.	Prot.	Carb.	Fat	Chol.	Sod.	Fiber
Cookies, chocolate wafers 1 oz (28g)	121	35	2	20	4	1	162	0.8
Cookies, coconut macaroons, prepared from recipe 1 medium cookie (2″ dia) (24g)	97	0	1	17	3	0	59	0.5
Cookies, fig bars 1 oz (28g)	97	17	1	20	2	0	98	1.4
Cookies, fortune 1 cookie (8g)	30	2	0	7	0	1	22	0.2
Cookies, fudge, cake-type (includes trolley cakes) 1 cookie (21g)	73	7	1	16	1	0	40	0.6
Cookies, gingersnaps 1 cookie (7g)	29	6	0	5	1	0	46	0.1
Cookies, graham crackers, chocolate-coated 1 cracker ($2\frac{1}{2}$″ square) (14g)	68	28	1	9	3	0	41	0.4
Cookies, graham crackers, plain or honey (includes cinnamon) 1 oz (28g)	118	25	2	22	3	0	169	0.8
Cookies, ladyfingers, with lemon juice and rind 1 anisette sponge ($4″ \times 1\frac{1}{8}″ \times \frac{7}{8}″$)	47	0	1	8	1	47	19	0.1
Cookies, ladyfingers, without lemon juice and rind 1 anisette sponge ($4″ \times 1\frac{1}{8}″ \times \frac{7}{8}″$)	47	0	1	8	1	47	19	
Cookies, marshmallow, chocolate-coated (includes marshmallow pies) 1 oz (28g)	118	42	1	19	5	0	47	0.6
Cookies, molasses 1 oz (28g)	120	32	2	21	4	0	129	0.3
Cookies, oatmeal, commercially prepared, fat-free 1 oz (28g)	91	5	2	22	1	0	83	2.0
Cookies, oatmeal, commercially prepared 1 big cookie ($3\frac{1}{2}″$ - 4″ dia)	113	40	2	17	5	0	96	0.8
Cookies, oatmeal, commercially prepared, soft-type 1 cookie (15g)	61	20	1	10	2	1	52	0.4

Food Serving size	Cal.	Fat cal.	Prot.	Carb.	Fat	Chol.	Sod.	Fiber
Cookies, oatmeal, commercially prepared, special dietary 1 medium cookie ($1\frac{5}{8}''$ dia) (7g)	31	11	0	5	1	0	1	0.2
Cookies, oatmeal, prepared from recipe, with raisins 1 cookie ($2\frac{5}{8}''$ dia) (15g)	65	0	1	10	2	5	81	
Cookies, oatmeal, prepared from recipe, without raisins 1 cookie ($2\frac{5}{8}''$ dia) (15g)	67	0	1	10	3	5	90	
Cookies, oatmeal, refrigerated dough, baked 1 cookie (12g)	57	0	1	8	3	3	39	0.4
Cookies, peanut butter sandwich 1 cookie (14g)	67	25	1	9	3	0	52	0.3
Cookies, peanut butter sandwich, special dietary 1 cookie (10g)	54	30	1	5	3	0	41	
Cookies, peanut butter, commercially prepared 1 cookie (15g)	72	31	2	9	4	0	62	0.3
Cookies, peanut butter, commercially prepared, soft-type 1 cookie (15g)	69	31	1	9	4	0	50	0.3
Cookies, peanut butter, prepared from recipe 1 cookie (3″ dia) (20g)	95	0	2	12	5	6	104	
Cookies, peanut butter, refrigerated dough, baked 1 cookie (12g)	60	0	1	7	3	4	52	0.1
Cookies, raisin, soft-type 1 cookie (15g)	60	18	1	10	2	0	51	0.2
Cookies, shortbread, commercially prepared, pecan 1 cookie (2″ dia) (14g)	76	39	1	8	4	5	39	0.3
Cookies, shortbread, commercially prepared, plain 1 cookie ($1\frac{5}{8}''$ square) (8g)	40	17	0	5	2	2	36	0.2
Cookies, shortbread, prepared from recipe, made with butter 1 medium cookie ($1\frac{1}{2}''$ dia) (11g)	60	0	1	6	4	10	51	

Food Serving size	Cal.	Fat cal.	Prot.	Carb.	Fat	Chol.	Sod.	Fiber
Cookies, shortbread, prepared from recipe, made with margarine 1 medium cookie $(1\frac{1}{2}''$ dia) (11g)	60	0	1	6	4	0	56	
Cookies, sugar wafers with creme filling 1 large wafer $(3\frac{1}{2}'' \times 1'' \times \frac{1}{2}'')$ (9g)	46	19	0	6	2	0	13	0.1
Cookies, sugar wafers with creme filling, special dietary 1 wafer (4g)	20	9	0	3	1	0	0	
Cookies, sugar, commercially prepared (includes vanilla) 1 cookie (15g)	72	28	1	10	3	8	54	0.2
Cookies, sugar, commercially prepared, special dietary 1 medium cookie $(1\frac{5}{8}''$ dia) (7g)	30	8	0	5	1	0	0	0.1
Cookies, sugar, prepared from recipe, made with butter 1 cookie (3″ dia) (14g)	66	0	1	8	3	12	64	
Cookies, sugar, prepared from recipe, made with margarine 1 cookie (3″ dia) (14g)	66	0	1	8	3	4	69	0.1
Cookies, sugar, refrigerated dough, baked 1 cookie (12g)	58	0	1	8	3	4	56	0.1
Cookies, vanilla sandwich with creme filling 1 oval cookie $(3\frac{1}{8}'' \times 1\frac{1}{4}'' \times \frac{3}{8}'')$	72	26	1	11	3	0	52	0.3
Cookies, vanilla wafers, higher fat 1 wafer (6g)	28	10	0	4	1	0	18	0.1
Cookies, vanilla wafers, lower fat 1 oz (28g)	123	37	1	21	4	16	87	0.6

Crackers

Cracker meal 1 oz (28g)	107	5	3	23	1	0	8	0.8
Crackers, cheese, low sodium 1 cup (62g)	312		6	36	16	8	284	1.2
Crackers, cheese 1 cup, bite size (62g)	312	136	6	36	16	8	617	1.2

Food Serving size	Cal.	Fat cal.	Prot.	Carb.	Fat	Chol.	Sod.	Fiber
Crackers, cheese, sandwich-type with peanut butter filling								
1 sandwich (7g)	34	14	1	4	2	0	69	0.2
Crackers, crispbread, rye								
1 crispbread or cracker								
(10g)	37	1	1	8	0	0	26	1.6
Crackers, matzo, egg and onion								
$\frac{1}{2}$oz (14g)	55	5	1	11	1	7	40	0.7
Crackers, matzo, egg								
$\frac{1}{2}$oz (14g)	55	2	2	11	0	12	3	0.4
Crackers, matzo, plain								
$\frac{1}{2}$oz (14g)	55	1	1	12	0	0	0	0.4
Crackers, matzo, whole-wheat								
$\frac{1}{2}$oz (14g)	49	2	2	11	0	0	0	1.7
Crackers, Melba toast, plain, without salt								
1 cup, pieces (30g)	117	8	4	23	1	0	6	1.8
Crackers, Melba toast, plain								
1 cup, pieces (30g)	117	8	4	23	1	0	249	1.8
Crackers, Melba toast, rye (includes pumpernickel)								
1 toast (5g)	19	1	1	4	0	0	45	0.4
Crackers, Melba toast, wheat								
1 toast (5g)	19	1	1	4	0	0	42	0.3
Crackers, milk								
1 cracker (11g)	50	15	1	8	2	2	65	0.2
Crackers, rusk toast								
1 rusk (10g)	41	6	1	7	1	3	25	
Crackers, rye, sandwich-type with cheese filling								
1 sandwich cracker (7g)	34	14	1	4	2	1	73	0.3
Crackers, rye, wafers, plain								
1 cracker								
$(4\frac{1}{2}'' \times 2\frac{1}{2}'' \times \frac{1}{8}'')$								
(11g)	37	1	1	9	0	0	87	2.5
Crackers, rye, wafers, seasoned								
$\frac{1}{2}$oz (14g)	53	11	1	10	1	0	124	2.9

Food Serving size	Cal.	Fat cal.	Prot.	Carb.	Fat	Chol.	Sod.	Fiber
Crackers, saltines (includes oyster, soda, soup) 1 cup, oyster crackers (45g)	195	48	4	32	5	0	586	1.4
Crackers, saltines, fat-free, low-sodium 3 saltines (15g)	59	3	2	12	0	0	95	0.4
Crackers, saltines, low salt (includes oyster, soda, soup) 1 cracker (3g)	13	3	0	2	0	0	19	0.1
Crackers, saltines, unsalted tops (includes oyster, soda, soup) 1 cracker (3g)	13	3	0	2	0	0	23	0.1
Crackers, standard snack-type, low salt 1 cup, bite size (62g)	311	136	4	38	16	0	231	1.2
Crackers, standard snack-type 1 cup, bite size (62g)	311	136	4	38	16	0	525	1.2
Crackers, standard snack-type, sandwich, with cheese filling 1 sandwich cracker (7g)	33	13	1	4	1	0	98	0.1
Crackers, standard snack-type, sandwich, with peanut butter filling 1 sandwich cracker (7g)	34	14	1	4	2	0	66	0.2
Crackers, wheat, low salt 1 cup, crushed (3g)	14	6	0	2	1	0	8	0.1
Crackers, wheat 1 Euphrates (4g)	19	7	0	3	1	0	32	0.2
Crackers, wheat, sandwich, with cheese filling 1 sandwich cracker (7g)	35	15	1	4	2	0	64	0.2
Crackers, wheat, sandwich, with peanut butter filling 1 sandwich cracker (7g)	35	16	1	4	2	0	56	0.3
Crackers, whole-wheat, low salt 1 cracker (4g)	18	6	0	3	1	0	10	0.4
Crackers, whole-wheat 1 cracker (4g)	18	6	0	3	1	0	26	0.4

Croissants

Food Serving size	Cal.	Fat cal.	Prot.	Carb.	Fat	Chol.	Sod.	Fiber
Croissants, apple 1 oz (28g)	71	22	2	10	3	14	77	0.6
Croissants, butter 1 oz (28g)	114	52	2	13	6	21	208	0.8

Food Serving size	Cal.	Fat cal.	Prot.	Carb.	Fat	Chol.	Sod.	Fiber
Croissants, cheese								
1 oz (28g)	116	52	3	13	6	18	155	0.8

English Muffins

English muffins, mixed-grain (includes granola)								
1 oz (28g)	66	5	3	13	1	0	116	0.8
English muffins, mixed-grain, toasted (includes granola)								
1 oz (28g)	71	0	3	14	1	0	127	0.8
English muffins, plain, enriched, with calcium propionate (includes sourdough)								
1 oz (28g)	66	5	2	13	1	0	130	0.8
English muffins, plain, enriched, without calcium propionate(includes sourdough)								
1 oz (28g)	66	5	2	13	1	0	130	0.8
English muffins, plain, toasted, enriched, with calcium propionate (includes sourdough)								
1 oz (28g)	71	0	2	14	1	0	141	0.8
English muffins, plain, toasted, enriched, without calcium propionate (includes sourdough)								
1 oz (28g)	71	0	2	14	1	0	141	0.8
English muffins, plain, toasted, unenriched, with calcium propionate (includes sourdough)								
1 oz (28g)	71	0	2	14	1	0	141	
English muffins, plain, toasted, unenriched, without calcium propionate (includes sourdough)								
1 oz (28g)	71	0	2	14	1	0	141	
English muffins, plain, unenriched, with calcium propionate (includes sourdough)								
1 oz (28g)	66	5	2	13	1	0	130	
English muffins, plain, unenriched, without calcium propionate (includes sourdough)								
1 oz (28g)	66	5	2	13	1	0	130	
English muffins, raisin-cinnamon (includes apple-cinnamon)								
1 oz (28g)	68	7	2	14	1	0	125	0.8
English muffins, raisin-cinnamon, toasted (includes apple-cinnamon)								
1 oz (28g)	74	0	2	15	1	0	136	0.8

Food Serving size	Cal.	Fat cal.	Prot.	Carb.	Fat	Chol.	Sod.	Fiber
English muffins, wheat, toasted 1 oz (28g)	68	0	3	14	1	0	116	1.4
English muffins, wheat 1 oz (28g)	62	5	3	13	1	0	107	1.4
English muffins, whole-wheat, toasted 1 oz (28g)	62	0	3	12	1	0	194	2.0
English muffins, whole-wheat 1 oz (28g)	57	5	3	11	1	0	178	2.0

French Toast, Pancakes and Waffles

Food Serving size	Cal.	Fat cal.	Prot.	Carb.	Fat	Chol.	Sod.	Fiber
French toast, frozen, ready-to-heat 1 oz (28g)	60	15	2	9	2	23	139	0.3
French toast, prepared from recipe, made with low fat (2%) milk 1 oz (28g)	64	0	2	7	3	32	134	
French toast, prepared from recipe, made with whole milk 1 oz (28g)	65	0	2	7	3	33	134	
Pancakes plain, frozen, ready-to-heat (includes buttermilk) 1 oz (28g)	64	7	1	12	1	3	143	0.6
Pancakes, blueberry, prepared from recipe 1 oz (28g)	62	0	2	8	3	16	115	
Pancakes, buckwheat, dry mix, incomplete, prepared 1 oz (28g)	58	0	2	8	2	18	149	0.6
Pancakes, buttermilk, prepared from recipe 1 oz (28g)	64	0	2	8	3	16	146	
Pancakes, plain, dry mix, incomplete, prepared 1 oz (28g)	61	0	2	8	2	20	141	0.6
Pancakes, plain, prepared from recipe 1 oz (28g)	64	0	2	8	3	17	123	
Pancakes, special dietary, dry mix, prepared 1 pancake (3″ dia) (22g)	44	0	1	9	0	0	58	
Pancakes, whole-wheat, dry mix, incomplete, prepared 1 oz (28g)	58	0	2	8	2	17	160	0.8
Waffles, buttermilk, prepared from recipe 1 oz (28g)	81	0	2	9	4	19	168	

Food Serving size	Cal.	Fat cal.	Prot.	Carb.	Fat	Chol.	Sod.	Fiber
Waffles, plain, frozen, ready-to-heat (includes buttermilk)								
1 oz (28g)	70	20	2	11	2	6	209	0.6
Waffles, plain, frozen, ready-to-heat, toasted (includes buttermilk)								
1 oz (28g)	74	0	2	11	2	7	220	0.6
Waffles, plain, prepared from recipe								
1 oz (28g)	81	0	2	9	4	19	143	

Muffins

Food Serving size	Cal.	Fat cal.	Prot.	Carb.	Fat	Chol.	Sod.	Fiber
Muffins, blueberry, commercially prepared 1 miniature muffin								
$(1\frac{1}{4}''$ dia) (11g)	30	6	1	5	1	3	49	0.3
Muffins, blueberry, dry mix, prepared								
1 oz (28g)	84	0	1	14	3	13	122	0.3
Muffins, blueberry, prepared from recipe, made with low fat (2%) milk								
1 oz (28g)	80	0	2	11	3	10	123	
Muffins, blueberry, prepared from recipe, made with whole milk								
1 oz (28g)	81	0	2	11	3	11	123	
Muffins, blueberry, toaster-type, toasted								
1 oz (28g)	93	0	1	16	3	1	143	0.6
Muffins, blueberry, toaster-type								
1 oz (28g)	88	25	1	15	3	1	134	0.6
Muffins, corn, commercially prepared								
1 oz (28g)	85	20	2	14	2	14	146	0.8
Muffins, corn, prepared from recipe, made with low fat (2%) milk								
1 oz (28g)	88	0	2	12	3	12	164	
Muffins, corn, prepared from recipe, made with whole milk								
1 oz (28g)	90	0	2	12	4	13	164	
Muffins, corn, toaster-type, toasted								
1 oz (28g)	103	0	2	17	3	1	128	0.6
Muffins, corn, toaster-type								
1 oz (28g)	97	27	1	16	3	1	120	0.6
Muffins, oat bran								
1 oz (28g)	76	17	2	13	2	0	110	1.4

Food Serving size	Cal.	Fat cal.	Prot.	Carb.	Fat	Chol.	Sod.	Fiber
Muffins, plain, prepared from recipe, made with low fat (2%) milk								
1 oz (28g)	83	0	2	11	3	11	131	0.8
Muffins, plain, prepared from recipe, made with whole milk								
1 oz (28g)	84	0	2	11	3	12	131	0.8
Muffins, wheat bran, dry mix, prepared								
1 oz (28g)	77	0	2	13	3	19	131	1.1
Muffins, wheat bran, prepared from recipe, made with low fat (2%) milk								
1 oz (28g)	79	0	2	12	3	9	165	
Muffins, wheat bran, prepared from recipe, made with whole milk								
1 oz (28g)	81	0	2	12	4	10	165	
Muffins, wheat bran, toaster-type with raisins, toasted								
1 oz (28g)	88	0	2	16	3	3	148	2.2
Muffins, wheat bran, toaster-type with raisins								
1 oz (28g)	83	22	1	15	3	3	139	2.2

Pastries

Food Serving size	Cal.	Fat cal.	Prot.	Carb.	Fat	Chol.	Sod.	Fiber
Cream puffs, prepared from recipe, shell (includes eclair)								
1 oz (28g)	101	0	3	6	7	55	156	0.3
Cream puffs, prepared from recipe, shell, with custard filling								
1 oz (28g)	72	0	2	6	4	38	95	0.0
Danish pastry, cheese								
1 oz (28g)	105	54	2	10	6	13	126	0.3
Danish pastry, cinnamon, enriched								
1 oz (28g)	113	54	2	13	6	8	104	0.3
Danish pastry, cinnamon, unenriched								
1 oz (28g)	113	54	2	13	6	8	104	0.3
Danish pastry, fruit, enriched (includes apple, cinnamon, raisin, lemon, raspberry, strawberry)								
1 oz (28g)	104	44	1	13	5	6	99	0.6
Danish pastry, fruit, unenriched (includes apple, cinnamon, raisin, lemon, raspberry, strawberry)								
1 oz (28g)	104	44	1	13	5	6	99	0.6
Danish pastry, lemon, unenriched								
1 oz (28g)	104	44	1	13	5	6	99	0.6

Food Serving size	Cal.	Fat cal.	Prot.	Carb.	Fat	Chol.	Sod.	Fiber
Danish pastry, nut (includes almond, raisin nut, cinnamon nut)								
1 oz (28g)	120	61	2	13	7	13	102	0.6
Danish pastry, raspberry, unenriched								
1 oz (28g)	104	44	1	13	5	6	99	0.6
Doughnuts, cake-type, chocolate, sugared or glazed								
1 oz (28g)	117	49	1	16	6	16	95	0.6
Doughnuts, cake-type, plain (includes unsugared, old-fashioned)								
1 oz (28g)	118	57	1	14	6	10	153	0.6
Doughnuts, cake-type, plain, chocolate-coated or frosted								
1 oz (28g)	133	76	1	13	9	16	120	0.6
Doughnuts, cake-type, plain, sugared or glazed								
1 oz (28g)	119	57	1	14	6	9	113	0.6
Doughnuts, cake-type, wheat, sugared or glazed								
1 oz (28g)	101	47	2	12	5	6	99	0.6
Doughnuts, French crullers, glazed								
1 oz (28g)	115	44	1	17	5	3	97	0.3
Doughnuts, yeast-leavened, glazed, enriched (includes honey buns)								
1 doughnut hole (13g)	52	26	1	6	3	1	44	0.1
Doughnuts, yeast-leavened, glazed, unenriched (includes honey buns)								
1 oz (28g)	113	57	2	12	6	2	96	0.6
Doughnuts, yeast-leavened, with creme filling								
1 oz (28g)	101	59	2	8	7	7	87	0.3
Doughnuts, yeast-leavened, with jelly filling								
1 oz (28g)	95	47	2	11	5	7	82	0.3
Eclairs, custard-filled with chocolate glaze, prepared from recipe								
1 oz (28g)	73	0	2	7	4	36	94	0.3
Puff pastry, frozen, ready-to-bake, baked								
1 oz (28g)	156	0	2	13	11	0	71	0.3
Puff pastry, frozen, ready-to-bake								
1 oz (28g)	154	0	2	13	11	0	70	0.3
Strudel, apple								
1 oz (28g)	77	27	1	11	3	8	75	0.6
Sweet rolls, cheese								
1 oz (28g)	101	44	2	12	5	16	100	0.3

Food Serving size	Cal.	Fat cal.	Prot.	Carb.	Fat	Chol.	Sod.	Fiber
Sweet rolls, cinnamon, commercially prepared with raisins								
1 oz (28g)	104	39	2	14	4	18	107	0.6
Sweet rolls, cinnamon, refrigerated dough with frosting, baked								
1 oz (28g)	101	0	1	16	4	0	233	
Sweet rolls, prepared from recipe with raisins and nuts								
1 oz (28g)	96	0	2	15	4	6	91	
Toaster pastries, brown-sugar-cinnamon								
1 oz (28g)	115	34	1	19	4	0	119	0.3
Toaster pastries, fruit (includes apple, blueberry, cherry, strawberry)								
1 oz (28g)	110	25	1	20	3	0	117	0.6

Pies

Food Serving size	Cal.	Fat cal.	Prot.	Carb.	Fat	Chol.	Sod.	Fiber
Pie crust, cookie-type, prepared from recipe, chocolate wafer, baked								
$\frac{1}{8}$ of 9″ crust (27g)	139	0	1	15	9	1	185	
Pie crust, cookie-type, prepared from recipe, chocolate wafer, chilled								
$\frac{1}{8}$ of 9″ crust (28g)	142	0	1	15	9	0	188	0.6
Pie crust, cookie-type, prepared from recipe, graham cracker, baked								
1 tart shell (22g)	109	0	1	14	6	0	126	0.4
Pie crust, cookie-type, prepared from recipe, graham cracker, chilled								
$\frac{1}{8}$ of 9″ crust (30g)	145	0	1	19	7	0	168	0.6
Pie crust, cookie-type, prepared from recipe, vanilla wafer, baked								
$\frac{1}{8}$ of 9″ crust (22g)	119	0	1	11	8	9	116	
Pie crust, cookie-type, prepared from recipe, vanilla wafer, chilled								
1 cup (129g)	685	0	5	65	46	50	664	0.0
Pie crust, standard-type, dry mix, prepared, baked								
$\frac{1}{8}$ of 9″ crust (20g)	100	0	1	10	6	0	146	0.4
Pie crust, standard-type, frozen, ready-to-bake, baked								
$\frac{1}{8}$ of 9″ crust (16g)	82	0	1	8	5	0	104	0.2
Pie crust, standard-type, prepared from recipe, baked								
$\frac{1}{8}$ of 9″ crust (23g)	121	0	1	11	8	0	125	0.5
Pie, apple, commercially prepared, enriched flour								
1 oz (28g)	66	27	1	10	3	0	74	0.6
Pie, apple, commercially prepared, unenriched flour								
1 oz (28g)	66	27	1	10	3	0	74	0.6

Food Serving size	Cal.	Fat cal.	Prot.	Carb.	Fat	Chol.	Sod.	Fiber
Pie, apple, prepared from recipe								
1 oz (28g)	74	0	1	10	3	0	59	
Pie, banana cream, prepared from mix, no-bake type								
1 oz (28g)	70	32	1	9	4	8	81	0.3
Pie, banana cream, prepared from recipe								
1 oz (28g)	75	0	1	9	4	14	67	0.3
Pie, blueberry, commercially prepared								
1 oz (28g)	65	25	1	10	3	0	91	0.3
Pie, blueberry, prepared from recipe								
1 oz (28g)	69	0	1	10	3	0	52	
Pie, butterscotch, pudding-type, prepared from recipe								
1 oz (28g)	78	0	1	9	4	17	74	
Pie, cherry, commercially prepared								
1 oz (28g)	73	27	1	11	3	0	69	0.3
Pie, cherry, prepared from recipe								
1 oz (28g)	76	0	1	11	3	0	53	
Pie, chocolate cream, prepared from recipe								
1 oz (28g)	79	0	1	9	4	15	69	
Pie, chocolate creme, commercially prepared								
1 oz (28g)	85	47	1	10	5	1	38	0.6
Pie, chocolate mousse, prepared from mix, no-bake type								
1 oz (28g)	73	37	1	8	4	6	129	
Pie, coconut cream, prepared from mix, no-bake type								
1 oz (28g)	77	44	1	8	5	7	92	0.0
Pie, coconut cream, prepared from recipe								
1 oz (28g)	83	0	1	10	4	16	75	
Pie, coconut creme, commercially prepared								
1 oz (28g)	83	41	1	10	5	0	71	0.3
Pie, coconut custard, commercially prepared								
1 oz (28g)	73	32	2	8	4	10	94	0.6
Pie, egg custard, commercially prepared								
1 oz (28g)	59	30	2	6	3	9	67	0.6
Pie, egg custard, prepared from recipe								
1 oz (28g)	58	0	1	8	3	19	57	

Food Serving size	Cal.	Fat cal.	Prot.	Carb.	Fat	Chol.	Sod.	Fiber
Pie, fried pies, cherry 1 oz (28g)	88	39	1	12	4	0	105	0.8
Pie, fried pies, fruit 1 oz (28g)	88	39	1	12	4	0	105	0.8
Pie, fried pies, lemon 1 oz (28g)	88	39	1	12	4	0	105	0.8
Pie, lemon meringue, commercially prepared 1 oz (28g)	75	22	1	13	3	13	41	0.3
Pie, lemon meringue, prepared from recipe 1 oz (28g)	80	0	1	11	4	15	68	
Pie, mince, prepared from recipe 1 oz (28g)	81	0	1	13	3	0	71	0.8
Pie, peach 1 oz (28g)	62	25	1	9	3	0	76	0.3
Pie, pecan, commercially prepared 1 oz (28g)	112	44	1	16	5	9	119	1.1
Pie, pecan, prepared from recipe 1 oz (28g)	115	0	1	15	6	24	73	
Pie, pumpkin, commercially prepared 1 oz (28g)	59	25	1	8	3	6	79	0.8
Pie, pumpkin, prepared from recipe 1 oz (28g)	57	0	1	7	3	12	63	
Pie, vanilla cream, prepared from recipe 1 oz (28g)	78	0	1	9	4	17	73	0.3

Rolls

Food Serving size	Cal.	Fat cal.	Prot.	Carb.	Fat	Chol.	Sod.	Fiber
Rolls, dinner, egg 1 oz (28g)	86	15	3	15	2	14	153	1.1
Rolls, dinner, oat bran 1 oz (28g)	66	12	3	11	1	0	116	1.1
Rolls, dinner, plain, commercially prepared (includes brown-and-serve) 1 hamburger, frankfurter, onion roll	129	26	3	22	3	0	224	1.3

Rolls, dinner, plain, prepared from recipe, made with low fat (2%) milk

Food Serving size	Cal.	Fat cal.	Prot.	Carb.	Fat	Chol.	Sod.	Fiber
1 oz (28g)	88	0	2	15	2	10	116	0.6
Rolls, dinner, plain, prepared from recipe, made with whole milk								
1 oz (28g)	90	0	2	15	2	10	116	
Rolls, dinner, rye								
1 medium (36g)	103	9	4	19	1	0	321	1.8
Rolls, dinner, wheat								
1 roll (1 oz) (28g)	76	15	3	13	2	0	95	1.1
Rolls, dinner, whole-wheat								
1 hamburger, frankfurter roll (43g)	114	0	4	22	2	0	206	3.4
Rolls, French								
1 oz (28g)	78	10	3	14	1	0	171	0.8
Rolls, hamburger or hot dog, mixed-grain								
1 oz (28g)	74	15	3	13	2	0	128	1.1
Rolls, hamburger or hot dog, plain								
1 oz (28g)	80	12	2	14	1	0	157	0.8
Rolls, hamburger or hot dog, reduced-calorie								
1 oz (28g)	55	5	2	12	1	0	124	1.7
Rolls, hard (includes kaiser)								
1 oz (28g)	82	10	3	15	1	0	152	0.6

Miscellaneous Baked Goods

Food Serving size	Cal.	Fat cal.	Prot.	Carb.	Fat	Chol.	Sod.	Fiber
Croutons, plain								
$\frac{1}{2}$ oz (14g)	57	9	2	10	1	0	98	0.7
Croutons, seasoned								
1 fast food package (10g)	47	16	1	6	2	0	124	0.5
Hush puppies, prepared from recipe								
1 oz (28g)	94	0	2	13	4	13	187	0.8
Ice cream cones, cake or wafer-type								
1 cone (4g)	17	2	0	3	0	0	6	0.1
Ice cream cones, sugar, rolled-type								
1 cone (10g)	40	4	1	8	0	0	32	0.2
Phyllo dough								
1 sheet dough (19g)	57	0	1	10	1	0	92	0.4

Food Serving size	Cal.	Fat cal.	Prot.	Carb.	Fat	Chol.	Sod.	Fiber
Popovers, dry mix, prepared 1 oz (28g)	57	0	2	9	1	31	122	
Popovers, prepared from recipe, made with low fat (2%) milk 1 oz (28g)	61	0	3	8	2	32	57	0.3
Popovers, prepared from recipe, made with whole milk 1 oz (28g)	63	0	3	8	2	33	57	
Taco shells, baked, without added salt 1 medium (approx 5″ dia) (13g)	61	26	1	8	3	0	2	1.0
Taco shells, baked 1 large ($6\frac{1}{2}$″ dia) (21g)	98	43	1	13	5	0	77	1.7
Tortillas, ready-to-bake or -fry, corn, without added salt 1 medium tortilla (approx 6″ dia) (26g)	58	4	2	12	1	0	3	1.3
Tortillas, ready-to-bake or -fry, corn 1 medium tortilla (approx 6″ dia) (26g)	58	4	2	12	1	0	42	1.3
Tortillas, ready-to-bake or -fry, flour 1 oz (28g)	91	17	3	16	2	0	134	0.8
Wonton wrappers (includes egg roll wrappers) 1 oz (28g)	81	0	3	16	1	3	160	0.6

Sausages and Luncheon Meats

Food Serving size	Cal.	Fat cal.	Prot.	Carb.	Fat	Chol.	Sod.	Fiber
Barbecue loaf, pork, beef 1 slice $(5\frac{7}{8}'' \times 3\frac{1}{2}'' \times \frac{1}{16}'')$ (23g)	40	19	4	1	2	9	307	0.0
Beef, cured, corned beef, canned 1 slice (.75 oz) (21g)	53	28	6	0	3	18	211	0.0
Beef, cured, dried beef 5 slices (21g)	35	8	6	0	1	9	729	0.0
Beef, cured, luncheon meat, jellied 1 slice (1 oz) $(4'' \times 4'' \times \frac{3}{32}'' \text{ thick})$	31	8	5	0	1	10	370	0.0
Beef, cured, pastrami 1 slice (1 oz) (28g)	98	73	5	1	8	26	344	0.0
Beef, cured, sausage, cooked, smoked 1 oz (28g)	87	68	4	1	8	19	317	0.0
Beef, cured, smoked, chopped beef 1 slice (1 oz) (28g)	37	10	6	1	1	13	352	0.0
Beef, cured, thin-sliced beef 5 slices (21g)	37	8	6	1	1	9	302	0.0
Beerwurst, beer salami, beef 1 slice, $(2\frac{3}{4}'' \text{ dia} \times \frac{1}{16}'')$ (6g)	20	16	1	0	2	4	62	0.0

Food Serving size	Cal.	Fat cal.	Prot.	Carb.	Fat	Chol.	Sod.	Fiber
Beerwurst, beer salami, pork 1 slice, ($2\frac{3}{4}''$ dia x $\frac{1}{16}''$) (6g)	14	10	1	0	1	4	74	0.0
Berliner, pork, beef 1 slice ($2\frac{1}{2}''$ dia x $\frac{1}{4}''$ thick) (23g)	53	35	3	1	4	11	298	0.0
Blood sausage 1 slice ($5'' \times 4\frac{5}{8}'' \times \frac{1}{16}''$) (25g)	95	77	4	0	9	30	170	0.0
Bologna, beef and pork 1 slice ($4''$ dia x $\frac{1}{8}''$ thick) (23g)	73	58	3	1	6	13	234	0.0
Bologna, beef 1 slice ($4''$ dia x $\frac{1}{8}''$ thick) (23g)	72	58	3	0	6	13	226	0.0
Bologna, pork 1 slice ($4''$ dia x $\frac{1}{8}''$ thick) (23g)	57	41	3	0	5	14	272	0.0
Bologna, turkey 1 oz (28g)	56	38	4	0	4	28	246	0.0
Bratwurst, cooked, pork 1 oz (28g)	84	66	4	1	7	17	156	0.0
Bratwurst, pork, beef, nonfat dry milk added 1 oz (28g)	90	71	4	1	8	18	311	0.0
Braunschweiger (a liver sausage), pork 1 slice ($2\frac{1}{2}''$ dia x $\frac{1}{4}''$ thick) (18g)	65	52	3	1	6	28	206	0.0
Cheesefurter, cheese smokie, pork, beef 1 oz (28g)	92	73	4	1	8	19	303	0.0

Food Serving size	Cal.	Fat cal.	Prot.	Carb.	Fat	Chol.	Sod.	Fiber
Chicken roll, light meat 2 slices (57g)	91	36	11	1	4	29	333	0.0
Chicken spread, canned 1 tablespoon (13g)	25	14	2	1	2	7	50	0.0
Chorizo, pork and beef 1 oz (28g)	127	96	7	1	11	25	346	0.0
Corned beef loaf, jellied 1 slice (1 oz) ($4''$ x $4''$ x $\frac{3}{32}''$ thick)	43	15	6	0	2	13	267	0.0
Dutch brand loaf, pork, beef 1 slice (1 oz) ($4''$ x $4''$ x $\frac{3}{32}''$ thick)	67	45	4	2	5	13	350	0.0
Frankfurter, beef and pork 1 frankfurter ($5''$ long x $\frac{3}{4}''$ dia	144	118	5	1	13	23	504	0.0
Frankfurter, beef 1 frankfurter ($5''$ long x $\frac{3}{4}''$ dia)	142	114	5	1	13	27	462	0.0
Frankfurter, chicken 1 oz (28g)	72	48	4	2	5	28	384	0.0
Frankfurter, turkey 1 oz (28g)	63	45	4	0	5	30	399	0.0
Ham, chopped, canned 1 slice ($4\frac{1}{4}''$ x $4\frac{1}{4}''$ x $\frac{1}{16}''$) (21g)	50	36	3	0	4	10	287	0.0
Ham, chopped, not canned 1 slice ($4\frac{1}{4}''$ x $4\frac{1}{4}''$ x $\frac{1}{16}''$) (21g)	48	32	4	0	4	11	288	0.0
Ham, minced 1 slice ($4\frac{1}{4}''$ x $4\frac{1}{4}''$ x $\frac{1}{16}''$) (21g)	55	40	3	0	4	15	261	0.0

Food Serving size	Cal.	Fat cal.	Prot.	Carb.	Fat	Chol.	Sod.	Fiber
Ham, sliced, extra lean (approximately 5% fat) 1 slice ($6\frac{1}{4}''$ x 4" x $\frac{1}{16}''$) (28g)	37	13	5	0	1	13	400	0.0
Ham, sliced, regular (approximately 11% fat) 1 slice ($6\frac{1}{4}''$ x 4" x $\frac{1}{16}''$) (28g)	51	28	5	1	3	16	369	0.0
Ham and cheese loaf or roll 1 slice (1 oz) (4" x 4" x $\frac{3}{32}''$ thick)	73	51	5	0	6	16	376	0.0
Ham and cheese spread 1 tablespoon (15g)	37	26	2	0	3	9	180	0.0
Ham salad spread 1 tablespoon (15g)	32	22	1	2	2	6	137	0.0
Headcheese, pork 1 slice (1 oz) (4" x 4" x $\frac{3}{32}''$ thick)	59	40	4	0	4	23	352	0.0
Honey loaf, pork, beef 1 slice (1 oz) (4" x 4" x $\frac{3}{32}''$ thick)	36	10	4	1	1	10	370	0.0
Honey roll sausage, beef 1 slice (4" dia x $\frac{1}{8}''$ thick) (23g)	42	21	4	0	2	12	304	0.0
Hot dog, *see* **Frankfurter**								
Italian sausage, pork 1 link, 5/lb (67g)	216	157	13	1	17	52	618	0.0
Kielbasa, kolbassy, pork, beef, nonfat dry milk added 1 slice (6" x $3\frac{3}{4}''$ x $\frac{1}{16}''$) (26g)	81	63	3	1	7	17	280	0.0
Knackwurst, knockwurst, pork, beef 1 oz (28g)	86	71	3	1	8	16	283	0.0

Food Serving size	Cal.	Fat cal.	Prot.	Carb.	Fat	Chol.	Sod.	Fiber
Lebanon bologna, beef 1 slice (4″ dia x $\frac{1}{8}$″ thick) (10 per 8-oz package	49	27	4	1	3	16	308	0.0
Liver cheese, pork 1 oz (28g)	85	66	4	1	7	49	343	0.0
Liver sausage, liverwurst, pork 1 slice ($2\frac{1}{2}$″ dia x $\frac{1}{4}$″ thick) (18g)	59	45	3	0	5	28	155	0.0
Luncheon meat, beef, loaved 1 slice (1 oz) (4″ x 4″ x $\frac{3}{32}$″ thick)	86	66	4	1	7	18	372	0.0
Luncheon meat, beef, thin sliced 5 slices (21g)	37	8	6	1	1	9	302	0.0
Luncheon meat, pork, beef 1 slice (1 oz) (28g)	99	81	4	1	9	15	362	0.0
Luncheon meat, pork, canned 1 slice ($4\frac{1}{4}$″ x $4\frac{1}{4}$″ x $\frac{1}{16}$″) (21g)	70	57	3	0	6	13	271	0.0
Luncheon sausage, pork and beef 1 slice (4″ dia x $\frac{1}{8}$″ thick) (23g)	60	44	3	0	5	15	272	0.0
Luxury loaf, pork 1 slice (1 oz) (4″ x 4″ x $\frac{3}{32}$″ thick)	39	13	5	1	1	10	343	0.0
Mortadella, beef, pork 1 slice (15 per 8 oz package) (15g)	47	34	2	0	4	8	187	0.0
Mother's loaf, pork 1 slice ($4\frac{1}{4}$″ x $4\frac{1}{4}$″ x $\frac{1}{16}$″) (21g)	59	42	3	2	5	9	237	0.0

Food Serving size	Cal.	Fat cal.	Prot.	Carb.	Fat	Chol.	Sod.	Fiber
New England brand sausage, pork, beef 1 slice (4" dia x $\frac{1}{8}$" thick) (23g)	37	17	4	1	2	11	281	0.0
Olive loaf, pork 1 slice (1 oz) (4" x 4" x $\frac{3}{32}$" thick)	66	40	3	3	4	11	416	0.0
Pastrami, turkey 2 slices (57g)	80	31	10	1	3	31	596	0.0
Pate, chicken liver, canned 1 tablespoon (13g)	26	15	2	1	2	51	50	0.0
Pate, goose liver, smoked, canned 1 tablespoon (13g)	60	52	1	1	6	20	91	0.0
Pate, liver, not specified, canned 1 tablespoon (13g)	41	33	2	0	4	33	91	0.0
Peppered loaf, pork, beef 1 slice (1 oz) (4" x 4" x $\frac{3}{32}$" thick)	41	15	5	1	2	13	426	0.0
Pepperoni, pork, beef 1 slice ($1\frac{3}{8}$" dia x $\frac{1}{8}$" thick) (6g)	30	24	1	0	3	5	122	0.0
Pickle and pimiento loaf, pork 1 slice (1 oz) (4" x 4" x $\frac{3}{32}$" thick)	73	53	3	2	6	10	389	0.0
Picnic loaf, pork, beef 1 slice (1 oz) (4" x 4" x $\frac{3}{32}$" thick)	65	43	4	1	5	11	326	0.0
Polish sausage, pork 1 oz (28g)	91	73	4	1	8	20	245	0.0
Pork and beef sausage, fresh, cooked 1 link (raw dimensions: 4" long x $\frac{7}{8}$")	51	42	2	0	5	9	105	0.0
Pork sausage, fresh, cooked 1 link (raw dimensions: 4" long x $\frac{7}{8}$")	48	36	3	0	4	11	168	0.0

Food Serving size	Cal.	Fat cal.	Prot.	Carb.	Fat	Chol.	Sod.	Fiber
Poultry salad sandwich spread 1 tablespoon (13g)	26	16	2	1	2	4	49	0.0
Salami, cooked, beef and pork 1 slice (4″ dia x $\frac{1}{8}$″ thick) (10 per 8-oz package	58	41	3	0	5	15	245	0.0
Salami, cooked, beef 1 slice (4″ dia x $\frac{1}{8}$″ thick) (10 per 8-oz package	60	44	3	1	5	15	270	0.0
Salami, cooked, turkey 2 slices (57g)	112	72	9	1	8	47	572	0.0
Salami, dry or hard, pork, beef 1 slice ($3\frac{1}{8}$″ dia x $\frac{1}{16}$″thick) (10g)	42	31	2	0	3	8	186	0.0
Salami, dry or hard, pork 1 slice ($3\frac{1}{8}$″ dia x $\frac{1}{16}$″thick) (10g)	41	31	2	0	3	8	226	0.0
Sandwich spread, pork, beef 1 tablespoon (15g)	35	23	1	2	3	6	152	0.0
Smoked link sausage, pork and beef, flour and nonfat dry milk added 1 little link (2″ long x $\frac{3}{4}$″ dia) (16g)	43	30	2	1	3	14	174	0.0
Smoked link sausage, pork and beef, nonfat dry milk added 1 little link (2″ long x $\frac{3}{4}$″ dia) (16g)	50	40	2	0	4	10	188	0.0
Smoked link sausage, pork and beef 1 little link (2″ long x $\frac{3}{4}$″ dia) (16g)	54	43	2	0	5	11	151	0.0

Food Serving size	Cal.	Fat cal.	Prot.	Carb.	Fat	Chol.	Sod.	Fiber
Smoked link sausage, pork 1 little link (2″ long x $\frac{3}{4}$″ dia) (16g)	62	46	4	0	5	11	240	0.0
Thuringer, cervelat, summer sausage, beef, pork 1 slice ($4\frac{1}{8}$″ dia x $\frac{1}{8}$″ thick)	77	62	4	0	7	17	286	0.0
Turkey breast meat 1 slice ($3\frac{1}{2}$″ square; 8 per 6-oz package)	23	4	5	0	0	9	301	0.0
Turkey ham, cured turkey thigh meat 2 slices (57g)	73	26	11	0	3	32	568	0.0
Turkey roll, light and dark meat 1 oz (28g)	42	18	5	1	2	15	164	0.0
Turkey roll, light meat 1 oz (28g)	41	18	5	0	2	12	137	0.0
Vienna sausage, canned, beef and pork 1 sausage ($\frac{7}{8}$″ dia x 2″ long) (16g)	45	36	2	0	4	8	152	0.0

Soups, Sauces, and Gravies

Food Serving size	Cal.	Fat cal.	Prot.	Carb.	Fat	Chol.	Sod.	Fiber
Gravies								
Gravy, au jus, dry 1 teaspoon (3g)	9	3	0	1	0	0	348	
Gravy, beef, canned 1 cup (233g)	123	42	9	12	5	7	1305	0.0
Gravy, chicken, canned 1 cup (238g)	188	127	5	12	14	5	1373	0.0
Gravy, mushroom, canned 1 cup (238g)	119	64	2	12	7	0	1357	0.0
Gravy, turkey, canned 1 tablespoon (15g)	8	3	0	1	0	0	87	0.0
Sauces								
Sauce, barbecue sauce 1 packet (9g)	7	2	0	1	0	0	73	0.1
Sauce, fish, ready-to-serve 1 tablespoon (18g)	6	0	1	1	0	0	1390	0.0
Sauce, hoisin, ready-to-serve 1 tablespoon (16g)	35	4	0	7	0	0	258	0.5
Sauce, homemade, white, medium $\frac{1}{2}$ cup (125g)	184	120	5	11	14	9	443	0.0

Food Serving size	Cal.	Fat cal.	Prot.	Carb.	Fat	Chol.	Sod.	Fiber
Sauce, homemade, white, thick $\frac{1}{2}$ cup (125g)	233	152	5	15	18	8	466	0.0
Sauce, homemade, white, thin $\frac{1}{2}$ cup (125g)	131	76	5	9	9	10	410	0.0
Sauce, oyster, ready-to-serve 1 tablespoon (4g)	2	0	0	0	0	0	109	0.0
Sauce, plum, ready-to-serve 1 tablespoon (19g)	35	2	0	8	0	0	102	0.2
Sauce, ready-to-serve, pepper or hot $\frac{1}{4}$ teaspoon (1g)	0	0	0	0	0	0	26	0.0
Sauce, ready-to-serve, pepper, TABASCO $\frac{1}{4}$ teaspoon (1g)	0	0	0	0	0	0	6	0.0
Sauce, ready-to-serve, salsa 1 tablespoon (16g)	4	0	0	1	0	0	41	0.3
Sauce, soy sauce 1 teaspoon (6g)	3	0	0	1	0	0	343	0.0

Soups

Food Serving size	Cal.	Fat cal.	Prot.	Carb.	Fat	Chol.	Sod.	Fiber
Soup, bean with bacon, dehydrated, prepared with water 1 fl oz (33g)	13	3	1	2	0	0	116	1.0
Soup, bean with frankfurters, canned, prepared with equal volume water, commercial 1 cup (8 fl oz) (250g)	188	67	10	23	8	13	1093	
Soup, bean with ham, canned, chunky, ready-to-serve, commercial 1 cup (8 fl oz) (243g)	231	87	12	27	10	22	972	12.1
Soup, bean with pork, canned, prepared with equal volume water, commercial 1 fl oz (32g)	22	6	1	3	1	0	120	1.0
Soup, beef broth or bouillon, powder, prepared with water 1 fl oz (prepared) (30g)	2	0	0	0	0	0	167	0.0
Soup, beef broth or bullion, canned, ready-to-serve 1 cup (240g)	17	0	2	0	0	0	782	0.0
Soup, beef broth, bouillon, consomme, prepared with equal volume water, commercial 1 cup (8 fl oz) (241g)	29	0	5	2	0	0	636	0.0

Food Serving size	Cal.	Fat cal.	Prot.	Carb.	Fat	Chol.	Sod.	Fiber
Soup, beef broth, cubed, prepared with water								
1 fl oz (30g)	1	0	0	0	0	0	144	0.0
Soup, beef mushroom, canned, prepared with equal volume water, commercial								
1 cup (8 fl oz) (244g)	73	22	5	7	2	7	942	0.0
Soup, beef noodle, canned, prepared with equal volume water, commercial								
1 fl oz (30g)	10	3	1	1	0	1	117	0.0
Soup, beef noodle, dehydrated, prepared with water								
1 fl oz (31g)	5	0	0	1	0	0	129	0.0
Soup, beef, canned, chunky, ready-to-serve								
1 cup (240g)	170	43	12	19	5	14	866	2.4
Soup, black bean, canned, prepared with equal volume water, commercial								
1 fl oz (31g)	15	3	1	2	0	0	150	0.6
Soup, cauliflower, dehydrated, prepared with water								
1 cup (8 fl oz) (256g)	69	23	3	10	3	0	842	
Soup, cheese, canned, prepared with equal volume milk, commercial								
1 cup (251g)	231	133	10	15	15	48	1019	0.0
Soup, cheese, canned, prepared with equal volume water, commercial								
1 cup (8 fl oz) (247g)	156	87	5	10	10	30	958	0.0
Soup, chicken broth cubes, dehydrated, prepared with water								
1 cube (6 fl oz prepared) (182g)	9	0	0	2	0	0	593	
Soup, chicken broth or bouillon, dehydrated, prepared with water								
1 fl oz (30g)	3	0	0	0	0	0	182	0.0
Soup, chicken broth, canned, prepared with equal volume water, commercial								
1 cup (240g)	38	22	5	0	2	0	763	0.0
Soup, chicken gumbo, canned, prepared with equal volume water, commercial								
1 fl oz (30g)	7	3	0	1	0	1	117	0.3
Soup, chicken mushroom, canned, prepared with equal volume water, commercial								
1 cup (8 fl oz) (244g)	132	88	5	10	10	10	942	0.0

Food Serving size	Cal.	Fat cal.	Prot.	Carb.	Fat	Chol.	Sod.	Fiber
Soup, chicken noodle, canned, chunky, ready-to-serve								
1 cup (240g)	175	43	12	17	5	19	850	4.8
Soup, chicken noodle, canned, prepared with equal volume water, commercial								
1 fl oz (30g)	9	3	1	1	0	1	138	0.0
Soup, chicken noodle, dehydrated, prepared with water								
1 cup (240g)	50	0	2	7	0	2	1222	0.0
Soup, chicken noodle, with meatballs, canned, chunky, ready-to-serve								
1 cup (8 fl oz) (248g)	99	22	7	7	2	10	1039	
Soup, chicken rice, canned, chunky, ready-to-serve								
1 cup (240g)	127	22	12	12	2	12	888	0.0
Soup, chicken rice, dehydrated, prepared with water								
1 fl oz (30g)	7	3	0	1	0	0	116	0.0
Soup, chicken vegetable, canned, chunky, ready-to-serve								
1 cup (8 fl oz) (240g)	166	42	12	19	5	17	1068	
Soup, chicken vegetable, canned, prepared with equal volume water, commercial								
1 fl oz (30g)	9	3	1	1	0	1	118	0.0
Soup, chicken vegetable, dehydrated, prepared with water 1 packet (6 fl oz)								
(188g)	38	0	2	6	0	2	605	
Soup, chicken with dumplings, canned, prepared with equal volume water, commercial								
1 fl oz (30g)	12	5	1	1	1	4	107	0.0
Soup, chicken with rice, canned, prepared with equal volume water, commercial								
1 fl oz (30g)	8	3	0	1	0	1	101	0.0
Soup, chili beef, canned, prepared with equal volume water, commercial								
1 fl oz (31g)	21	8	1	3	1	2	128	1.2
Soup, clam chowder, Manhattan style, canned, chunky, ready-to-serve								
1 fl oz (30g)	17	3	1	2	0	2	125	0.3

Food Serving size	Cal.	Fat cal.	Prot.	Carb.	Fat	Chol.	Sod.	Fiber
Soup, clam chowder, Manhattan, canned, prepared with equal volume water								
1 fl oz (30g)	10	3	0	2	0	0	71	0.3
Soup, clam chowder, New England, canned, prepared with equal volume milk, commercial								
1 cup (248g)	164	66	10	17	7	22	992	2.5
Soup, clam chowder, New England, canned, prepared with equal volume water, commercial								
1 fl oz (30g)	12	3	1	2	0	1	113	0.3
Soup, consomme with gelatin, dehydrated, prepared with water								
1 fl oz (31g)	2	0	0	0	0	0	411	0.0
Soup, crab, canned, ready-to-serve								
1 cup (8 fl oz) (244g)	76	22	5	10	2	10	1235	0.0
Soup, cream of asparagus, canned, prepared with equal volume water, commercial								
1 cup (8 fl oz) (244g)	85	43	2	10	5	5	981	0.0
Soup, cream of asparagus, dehydrated, prepared with water								
1 cup (8 fl oz) (251g)	58	22	3	10	3	0	801	
Soup, cream of celery, canned, prepared with equal volume milk, commercial								
1 cup (8 fl oz) (248g)	164	87	5	15	10	32	1009	0.0
Soup, cream of celery, canned, prepared with equal volume water, commercial								
1 cup (244g)	90	43	2	10	5	15	949	0.0
Soup, cream of celery, dehydrated, prepared with water								
1 cup (8 fl oz) (254g)	64	22	3	10	3	0	838	
Soup, cream of chicken, canned, prepared with equal volume water, commercial								
1 fl oz (30g)	14	8	0	1	1	1	121	0.0
Soup, cream of chicken, dehydrated, prepared with water								
1 fl oz (33g)	14	6	0	2	1	0	150	0.0
Soup, cream of chicken, prepared with equal volume milk, commercial								
1 fl oz (31g)	24	14	1	2	2	3	131	0.0
Soup, cream of mushroom, canned, prepared with equal volume milk, commercial								
1 cup (8 fl oz) (248g)	203	109	5	15	12	20	918	0.0

Food Serving size	Cal.	Fat cal.	Prot.	Carb.	Fat	Chol.	Sod.	Fiber
Soup, cream of mushroom, canned, prepared with equal volume water, commercial								
1 cup (244g)	129	86	2	10	10	2	881	0.0
Soup, cream of onion, canned, prepared with equal volume milk, commercial								
1 cup (8 fl oz) (248g)	186	87	7	17	10	32	1004	0.0
Soup, cream of onion, canned, prepared with equal volume water, commercial								
1 cup (8 fl oz) (244g)	107	43	2	12	5	15	927	0.0
Soup, cream of potato, canned, prepared with equal volume milk, commercial								
1 cup (8 fl oz) (248g)	149	65	5	17	7	22	1061	0.0
Soup, cream of potato, canned, prepared with equal volume water, commercial								
1 cup (8 fl oz) (244g)	73	21	2	12	2	5	1000	0.0
Soup, cream of shrimp, canned, prepared with equal volume milk, commercial								
1 fl oz (31g)	20	11	1	2	1	4	130	0.0
Soup, cream of shrimp, canned, prepared with equal volume water, commercial								
1 cup (244g)	90	43	2	7	5	17	976	0.0
Soup, cream of vegetable, dehydrated, prepared with water								
1 packet (6 fl oz prepared) (195g)	80	34	2	10	4	0	878	0.0
Soup, escarole, canned, ready-to-serve								
1 cup (8 fl oz) (248g)	27	22	2	2	2	2	3864	
Soup, gazpacho, canned, ready-to-serve								
1 cup (244g)	46	0	7	5	0	0	739	0.0
Soup, leek, dehydrated, prepared with water								
1 cup (254g)	71	22	3	10	3	3	965	2.5
Soup, lentil with ham, canned, ready-to-serve								
1 cup (8 fl oz) (248g)	139	22	10	20	2	7	1319	
Soup, minestrone, canned, chunky, ready-to-serve								
1 cup (240g)	127	21	5	22	2	5	864	4.8

Food Serving size	Cal.	Fat cal.	Prot.	Carb.	Fat	Chol.	Sod.	Fiber
Soup, minestrone, canned, prepared with equal volume water, commercial								
1 cup (8 fl oz) (241g)	82	21	5	12	2	2	911	0.0
Soup, minestrone, dehydrated, prepared with water								
1 cup (8 fl oz) (254g)	79	23	5	13	3	3	1026	
Soup, mushroom barley, canned, prepared with equal volume water, commercial								
1 cup (8 fl oz) (244g)	73	22	2	12	2	0	891	0.0
Soup, mushroom with beef stock, canned, prepared with equal volume water, commercial								
1 cup (8 fl oz) (244g)	85	44	2	10	5	7	969	0.0
Soup, mushroom, dehydrated, prepared with water								
1 packet (6 fl oz prepared) (194g)	74	35	2	8	4	0	782	0.0
Soup, onion, canned, prepared with equal volume water, commercial								
1 cup (241g)	58	20	5	7	2	0	1053	0.0
Soup, onion, dehydrated, prepared with water								
1 packet (6 fl oz prepared) (184g)	20	0	0	4	0	0	635	0.0
Soup, oxtail, dehydrated, prepared with water								
1 cup (244g)	68	22	2	10	2	2	1166	0.0
Soup, oyster stew, canned, prepared with equal volume milk, commercial								
1 cup (8 fl oz) (245g)	135	65	7	10	7	32	1041	0.0
Soup, oyster stew, canned, prepared with equal volume water, commercial								
1 cup (8 fl oz) (241g)	58	43	2	5	5	14	981	
Soup, pea, green, canned, prepared with equal volume milk, commercial								
1 cup (8 fl oz) (254g)	239	68	13	33	8	18	970	2.5
Soup, pea, green, canned, prepared with equal volume water, commercial								
1 cup (250g)	165	22	8	28	3	0	918	2.5
Soup, pea, green, mix, dehydrated, prepared with water								
1 packet (6 fl oz prepared) (206g)	101	18	6	16	2	2	927	2.1

Food Serving size	Cal.	Fat cal.	Prot.	Carb.	Fat	Chol.	Sod.	Fiber
Soup, pea, split with ham, canned, chunky, ready-to-serve								
1 cup (240g)	185	43	12	26	5	7	965	4.8
Soup, pea, split with ham, canned, prepared with equal volume water, commercial								
1 cup (8 fl oz) (253g)	190	45	10	28	5	8	1007	2.5
Soup, pepperpot, canned, prepared with equal volume water, commercial								
1 cup (8 fl oz) (241g)	104	43	7	10	5	10	971	0.0
Soup, scotch broth, canned, prepared with equal volume water, commercial								
1 cup (241g)	80	22	5	10	2	5	1012	0.0
Soup, shark fin, restaurant-prepared								
1 cup (216g)	99	39	6	9	4	4	1082	0.0
Soup, stock, fish, home-prepared								
1 cup (233g)	40	21	5	0	2	2	363	0.0
Soup, stockpot, canned, prepared with equal volume water, commercial								
1 cup (8 fl oz) (247g)	99	44	5	12	5	5	1047	
Soup, tomato beef with noodle, canned, prepared with equal volume water, commercial								
1 cup (244g)	139	44	5	22	5	5	917	2.4
Soup, tomato bisque, canned, prepared with equal volume milk, commercial								
1 cup (8 fl oz) (251g)	198	66	8	30	8	23	1109	0.0
Soup, tomato bisque, canned, prepared with equal volume water, commercial								
1 cup (8 fl oz) (247g)	124	22	2	25	2	5	1047	0.0
Soup, tomato rice, canned, prepared with equal volume water, commercial								
1 cup (247g)	119	22	2	22	2	2	815	2.5
Soup, tomato vegetable, dehydrated, prepared with water								
1 cup (241g)	53	0	2	10	0	0	1092	0.0
Soup, tomato, canned, prepared with equal volume milk, commercial								
1 cup (8 fl oz) (248g)	161	43	5	22	5	17	744	2.5

Food Serving size	Cal.	Fat cal.	Prot.	Carb.	Fat	Chol.	Sod.	Fiber
Soup, tomato, canned, prepared with equal volume water, commercial								
1 cup (8 fl oz) (244g)	85	21	2	17	2	0	695	0.0
Soup, tomato, dehydrated, prepared with water								
1 packet, prepared (199g)	78	17	2	14	2	0	708	0.0
Soup, turkey noodle, canned, prepared with equal volume water, commercial								
1 fl oz (30g)	8	3	1	1	0	1	100	0.0
Soup, turkey vegetable, canned, prepared with equal volume water, commercial								
1 fl oz (30g)	9	3	0	1	0	0	113	0.0
Soup, turkey, chunky, ready-to-serve								
1 cup (8 fl oz) (236g)	135	42	9	14	5	9	923	
Soup, vegetable beef, dehydrated, prepared with water								
1 cup (253g)	53	0	3	8	0	0	1002	0.0
Soup, vegetable beef, prepared with equal volume water, commercial								
1 cup (8 fl oz) (244g)	78	22	5	10	2	5	791	0.0
Soup, vegetable with beef broth, canned, prepared with equal volume water, commercial								
1 cup (8 fl oz) (241g)	82	22	2	12	2	2	810	0.0
Soup, vegetable, canned, chunky, ready-to-serve, commercial								
1 cup (240g)	122	43	2	19	5	0	1010	0.0
Soup, vegetarian vegetable, canned, prepared with equal volume water, commercial								
1 cup (241g)	72	20	2	12	2	0	822	0.0

Beverages

Food Serving size	Cal.	Fat cal.	Prot.	Carb.	Fat	Chol.	Sod.	Fiber

Alcoholic Beverages

Alcoholic beverage, beer, light
| 1 fl oz (30g) | 8 | 0 | 0 | 0 | 0 | 0 | 1 | 0.0 |

Alcoholic beverage, beer, regular
| 1 fl oz (30g) | 12 | 0 | 0 | 1 | 0 | 0 | 2 | 0.0 |

Alcoholic beverage, Bloody Mary, prepared-from-recipe
| 1 fl oz (30g) | 23 | 0 | 0 | 1 | 0 | 0 | 67 | 0.0 |

Alcoholic beverage, bourbon and soda, prepared from recipe
| 1 fl oz (29g) | 26 | 0 | 0 | 0 | 0 | 0 | 4 | 0.0 |

Alcoholic beverage, creme de menthe, 72 proof
| 1 fl oz (34g) | 126 | 0 | 0 | 14 | 0 | 0 | 2 | 0.0 |

Alcoholic beverage, daiquiri, canned
| 1 fl oz (30g) | 38 | 0 | 0 | 5 | 0 | 0 | 12 | 0.0 |

Alcoholic beverage, daiquiri, prepared-from-recipe
| 1 fl oz (30g) | 56 | 0 | 0 | 2 | 0 | 0 | 2 | 0.0 |

Alcoholic beverage, distilled, all (gin, rum, vodka, whiskey) 100 proof
| 1 fl oz (28g) | 83 | 0 | 0 | 0 | 0 | 0 | 0 | 0.0 |

Alcoholic beverage, distilled, all (gin, rum, vodka, whiskey) 80 proof
| 1 fl oz (28g) | 65 | 0 | 0 | 0 | 0 | 0 | 0 | 0.0 |

Alcoholic beverage, distilled, all (gin, rum, vodka, whiskey) 86 proof
| 1 fl oz (28g) | 70 | 0 | 0 | 0 | 0 | 0 | 0 | 0.0 |

Alcoholic beverage, distilled, all (gin, rum, vodka, whiskey) 90 proof
| 1 fl oz (28g) | 74 | 0 | 0 | 0 | 0 | 0 | 0 | 0.0 |

Food Serving size	Cal.	Fat cal.	Prot.	Carb.	Fat	Chol.	Sod.	Fiber
Alcoholic beverage, distilled, all (gin, rum, vodka, whiskey) 94 proof								
1 fl oz (28g)	77	0	0	0	0	0	0	0.0
Alcoholic beverage, distilled, gin, 90 proof								
1 fl oz (28g)	74	0	0	0	0	0	1	0.0
Alcoholic beverage, distilled, rum, 80 proof								
1 fl oz (28g)	65	0	0	0	0	0	0	0.0
Alcoholic beverage, distilled, vodka, 80 proof								
1 fl oz (28g)	65	0	0	0	0	0	0	0.0
Alcoholic beverage, distilled, whiskey, 86 proof								
1 fl oz (28g)	70	0	0	0	0	0	0	0.0
Alcoholic beverage, gin and tonic, prepared-from-recipe								
1 fl oz (30g)	23	0	0	2	0	0	1	0.0
Alcoholic beverage, liqueur, coffee with cream, 34 proof								
1 fl oz (31g)	101	44	1	7	5	5	29	0.0
Alcoholic beverage, liqueur, coffee, 53 proof								
1 fl oz (35g)	118	0	0	16	0	0	3	0.0
Alcoholic beverage, liqueur, coffee, 63 proof								
1 fl oz (35g)	108	0	0	11	0	0	3	0.0
Alcoholic beverage, Manhattan, prepared-from-recipe								
1 fl oz (28g)	63	0	0	1	0	0	1	0.0
Alcoholic beverage, martini, prepared-from-recipe								
1 fl oz (28g)	62	0	0	0	0	0	1	0.0
Alcoholic beverage, pina colada, canned								
1 fl oz (33g)	78	22	0	9	3	0	23	0.0
Alcoholic beverage, pina colada, prepared-from-recipe								
1 fl oz (31g)	58	0	0	9	1	0	2	0.3
Alcoholic beverage, screwdriver, prepared-from-recipe								
1 fl oz (30g)	25	0	0	3	0	0	0	0.0
Alcoholic beverage, tequila sunrise, canned								
1 fl oz (31g)	34	0	0	3	0	0	18	0.0
Alcoholic beverage, tequila sunrise, prepared-from-recipe								
1 fl oz (31g)	34	0	0	3	0	0	1	0.0
Alcoholic beverage, Tom Collins, prepared-from-recipe								
1 fl oz (30g)	17	0	0	0	0	0	5	0.0

Food Serving size	Cal.	Fat cal.	Prot.	Carb.	Fat	Chol.	Sod.	Fiber
Alcoholic beverage, whiskey sour, canned								
1 fl oz (31g)	37	0	0	4	0	0	14	0.0
Alcoholic beverage, whiskey sour, prepared with water, whiskey and powder mix								
1 fl oz (29g)	48	0	0	5	0	0	13	0.0
Alcoholic beverage, whiskey sour, prepared-from-recipe								
1 fl oz (30g)	41	0	0	2	0	0	3	0.0
Alcoholic beverage, wine, dessert, dry								
1 fl oz (30g)	38	0	0	1	0	0	3	0.0
Alcoholic beverage, wine, dessert, sweet								
1 fl oz (30g)	46	0	0	4	0	0	3	0.0
Alcoholic beverage, wine, table, all								
1 fl oz (30g)	21	0	0	0	0	0	2	0.0
Alcoholic beverage, wine, table, red								
1 fl oz (30g)	22	0	0	1	0	0	2	0.0
Alcoholic beverage, wine, table, rose								
1 fl oz (30g)	21	0	0	0	0	0	2	0.0
Alcoholic beverage, wine, table, white								
1 fl oz (30g)	20	0	0	0	0	0	2	0.0

Non-alcoholic Beverages

Food Serving size	Cal.	Fat cal.	Prot.	Carb.	Fat	Chol.	Sod.	Fiber
Beef broth and tomato juice, canned								
1 fl oz (30g)	11	0	0	2	0	0	39	0.0
Carbonated beverage, club soda								
1 fl oz (30g)	0	0	0	0	0	0	6	0.0
Carbonated beverage, cola								
1 fl oz (31g)	13	0	0	3	0	0	1	0.0
Carbonated beverage, cream soda								
1 fl oz (31g)	16	0	0	4	0	0	4	0.0
Carbonated beverage, ginger ale								
1 fl oz (30g)	10	0	0	3	0	0	2	0.0
Carbonated beverage, grape soda								
1 fl oz (31g)	13	0	0	3	0	0	5	0.0
Carbonated beverage, lemon-lime soda								
1 fl oz (31g)	12	0	0	3	0	0	3	0.0

Food Serving size	Cal.	Fat cal.	Prot.	Carb.	Fat	Chol.	Sod.	Fiber
Carbonated beverage, low calorie, cola or pepper-types, with sodium saccharin								
1 fl oz (30g)	0	0	0	0	0	0	5	0.0
Carbonated beverage, low calorie, cola, with aspartame and sodium saccharin								
1 fl oz (30g)	0	0	0	0	0	0	3	0.0
Carbonated beverage, low calorie, cola, with aspartame								
1 fl oz (30g)	0	0	0	0	0	0	2	0.0
Carbonated beverage, low calorie, other than cola or pepper, with sodium saccharin								
1 fl oz (30g)	0	0	0	0	0	0	5	0.0
Carbonated beverage, orange								
1 fl oz (31g)	15	0	0	4	0	0	4	0.0
Carbonated beverage, pepper-type								
1 fl oz (31g)	13	0	0	3	0	0	3	0.0
Carbonated beverage, root beer								
1 fl oz (31g)	13	0	0	3	0	0	4	0.0
Carbonated beverage, tonic water								
1 fl oz (30g)	10	0	0	3	0	0	1	0.0
Carob-flavor beverage mix, powder, prepared with milk								
1 cup (8 fl oz) (256g)	195	0	8	23	8	33	133	0.0
Carob-flavor beverage mix, powder								
1 tablespoon (12g)	45	0	0	11	0	0	12	1.0
Chocolate syrup, with added nutrients								
1 tablespoon (19g)	47	2	0	13	0	0	29	0.4
Chocolate syrup, without added nutrients								
1 tablespoon (19g)	41	2	0	11	0	0	18	0.4
Chocolate-flavor beverage mix, powder, prepared with milk								
1 cup (8 fl oz) (266g)	226	0	8	32	8	32	165	0.0
Chocolate-flavor beverage mix, powder 2–3 heaping teaspoons								
(22g)	77	6	1	20	1	0	46	1.3
Citrus fruit juice drink, frozen concentrate, prepared with water								
1 fl oz (31g)	14	0	0	4	0	0	1	0.0

Food Serving size	Cal.	Fat cal.	Prot.	Carb.	Fat	Chol.	Sod.	Fiber
Clam and tomato juice, canned								
1 fl oz (30g)	14	0	0	3	0	0	120	0.0
Cocoa mix, NESTLE, CARNATION Hot Cocoa Mix With Marshmallows								
1 envelope (28g)	112		1	24	1	2	96	0.6
Cocoa mix, NESTLE, CARNATION No Sugar Added Hot Cocoa Mix								
1 envelope (15g)	55		4	8	0	3	142	0.8
Cocoa mix, NESTLE, CARNATION Rich Chocolate Hot Cocoa Mix								
1 envelope (28g)	112		1	24	1	2	102	0.6
Cocoa mix, with added nutrients, powder, prepared with water 1 packet dry mix with 6								
fl oz water (209g)	119	0	2	25	2	0	207	0.0
Cocoa mix, with added nutrients, powder								
1 packet (1.1 oz) (31g)	119	27	2	24	3	1	200	0.9
Cocoa mix, without added nutrients, powder, prepared with water 1 oz packet with 6 fl oz								
water (206g)	103	0	4	23	2	2	148	2.1
Cocoa mix, without added nutrients, powder 1 serving (3 heaping teaspoons or 1								
envelope)	101	10	3	22	1	1	141	0.3
Coffee substitute, cereal grain beverage, powder, prepared with milk								
1 cup (6 fl oz) (185g)	120	0	6	11	6	24	91	0.0
Coffee substitute, cereal grain beverage, prepared with water								
1 fl oz (30g)	2	0	0	0	0	0	1	0.0
Coffee, brewed, espresso, restaurant-prepared								
100 grams	9	0	0	2	0	0	14	0.0
Coffee, brewed, prepared with tap water								
1 fl oz (30g)	1	0	0	0	0	0	1	0.0
Coffee, instant, decaffeinated, powder, prepared with water								
1 cup (6 fl oz) (179g)	4	0	0	0	0	0	5	0.0
Coffee, instant, regular, prepared with water								
1 fl oz (30g)	1	0	0	0	0	0	1	0.0
Coffee, instant, with chicory, prepared with water								
1 cup (6 fl oz) (179g)	7	0	0	2	0	0	11	0.0

Food Serving size	Cal.	Fat cal.	Prot.	Carb.	Fat	Chol.	Sod.	Fiber
Coffee, instant, with sugar, cappuccino-flavor, powder 2 teaspoons, rounded (14g)	61	18	0	11	2	0	97	0.0
Coffee, instant, with sugar, cappuccino-flavor, powder, prepared with water 1 cup (6 fl oz) (192g)	61	0	0	12	2	0	104	0.0
Coffee, instant, with sugar, French-flavor, powder, prepared with water 1 cup (6 fl oz) (189g)	57	0	0	8	4	0	30	0.0
Coffee, instant, with sugar, French-flavor, powder 2 teaspoons, rounded (12g)	60	31	0	7	4	0	25	0.0
Coffee, instant, with sugar, mocha-flavor, powder, prepared with water 1 cup (6 fl oz) (188g)	51	0	0	8	2	0	36	0.0
Coffee, instant, with sugar, mocha-flavor, powder 2 teaspoons, rounded (12g)	53	17	0	9	2	0	32	0.1
Cranberry juice cocktail, bottled 1 fl oz (32g)	18	0	0	4	0	0	1	0.0
Cranberry juice cocktail, frozen concentrate, prepared with water 1 fl oz (31g)	17	0	0	4	0	0	1	0.0
Cranberry-apple juice drink, bottled 1 fl oz (31g)	21	0	0	5	0	0	1	0.0
Cranberry-apricot juice drink, bottled 1 fl oz (31g)	20	0	0	5	0	0	1	0.0
Cranberry-grape juice drink, bottled 1 fl oz (31g)	17	0	0	4	0	0	1	0.0
Dairy drink mix, chocolate, reduced calorie, with aspartame, powder, prepared with water 6 fl oz (204g)	63	0	6	10	0	2	171	0.0
Dairy drink mix, chocolate, reduced calorie, with aspartame, powder 1 packet (.75 oz) (21g)	63	5	5	11	1	2	164	0.4
Eggnog-flavor mix, powder, prepared with milk 1 cup (8 fl oz) (272g)	261	0	8	38	8	33	163	0.0

Food Serving size	Cal.	Fat cal.	Prot.	Carb.	Fat	Chol.	Sod.	Fiber
Fruit punch drink, canned								
1 fl oz (31g)	15	0	0	4	0	0	7	0.0
Fruit punch drink, frozen concentrate, prepared with water								
1 fl oz (31g)	14	0	0	4	0	0	1	0.0
Fruit punch juice drink, frozen concentrate, prepared with water								
1 fl oz (31g)	16	0	0	4	0	0	2	0.0
Fruit punch-flavor drink, powder, with added sodium, prepared with water								
1 cup (8 fl oz) (262g)	97	0	0	26	0	0	37	0.0
Fruit punch-flavor drink, powder, without added sodium, prepared with water								
1 cup (8 fl oz) (262g)	97	0	0	26	0	0	10	0.0
Gelatin, drinking, orange-flavor, powder, prepared with water 1 packet, prepared								
(136g)	67	0	5	11	0	0	33	0.0
Gelatin, drinking, orange-flavor, powder								
1 packet (17g)	65	2	6	10	0	0	28	0.0
Grape drink, canned								
1 fl oz (31g)	14	0	0	4	0	0	2	0.0
Grape juice drink, canned								
1 fl oz (31g)	16	0	0	4	0	0	0	0.0
Lemonade, frozen concentrate, pink, prepared with water								
1 fl oz (31g)	12	0	0	3	0	0	1	0.0
Lemonade, frozen concentrate, white, prepared with water								
1 fl oz (31g)	12	0	0	3	0	0	1	0.0
Lemonade, low calorie, with aspartame, powder, prepared with water								
1 fl oz (30g)	1	0	0	0	0	0	1	0.0
Lemonade, powder, prepared with water								
1 cup (8 fl oz) (264g)	103	0	0	26	0	0	13	0.0
Lemonade-flavor drink, powder, prepared with water								
1 cup (8 fl oz) (266g)	112	0	0	29	0	0	19	0.0
Limeade, frozen concentrate, prepared with water								
1 can (1 oz) (31g)	13	0	0	3	0	0	1	0.0
Malt beverage								
1 fl oz (30g)	18	0	0	4	0	0	4	0.0

Food Serving size	Cal.	Fat cal.	Prot.	Carb.	Fat	Chol.	Sod.	Fiber
Malted milk-flavor mix, chocolate, added nutrients, powder, prepared with milk								
1 cup (8 fl oz) (265g)	225	0	8	29	8	34	244	0.0
Malted milk-flavor mix, chocolate, no added nutrients, powder, prepared with milk								
1 cup (8 fl oz) (265g)	228	0	8	29	8	34	172	0.0
Malted milk-flavor mix, natural, added nutrients, powder, prepared with milk								
1 cup (8 fl oz) (265g)	231	0	11	29	8	34	204	0.0
Malted milk-flavor mix, natural, no added nutrients, powder, prepared with milk								
1 cup (8 fl oz) (265g)	236	0	11	27	11	37	223	0.0
Orange and apricot juice drink, canned								
1 fl oz (31g)	16	0	0	4	0	0	1	0.0
Orange drink, breakfast type, with juice and pulp, frozen concentrate, prepared with water								
1 fl oz (31g)	14	0	0	3	0	0	3	0.0
Orange drink, canned								
1 fl oz (31g)	16	0	0	4	0	0	5	0.0
Orange-flavor drink, breakfast type, powder, prepared with water								
1 fl oz (31g)	14	0	0	4	0	0	2	0.0
Orange-flavor drink, breakfast type, with pulp, frozen concentrate, prepared with water								
1 fl oz (31g)	15	0	0	4	0	0	3	0.0
Pineapple and grapefruit juice drink, canned								
1 fl oz (31g)	15	0	0	4	0	0	4	0.0
Pineapple and orange juice drink, canned								
1 fl oz (31g)	16	0	0	4	0	0	1	0.0
Shake, fast food, chocolate								
1 fl oz (21g)	27	7	1	4	1	3	20	0.2
Shake, fast food, strawberry								
10 fl oz (283g)	320	75	8	54	8	31	235	0.0
Shake, fast food, vanilla								
1 fl oz (21g)	23	6	1	4	1	2	17	0.0

Food Serving size	Cal.	Fat cal.	Prot.	Carb.	Fat	Chol.	Sod.	Fiber
Strawberry-flavor beverage mix, powder, prepared with milk								
1 cup (8 fl oz) (266g)	234	0	8	32	8	32	128	0.0
Tea, brewed, prepared with tap water								
1 fl oz (30g)	0	0	0	0	0	0	1	0.0
Tea, herb, other than chamomile, brewed								
1 fl oz (30g)	0	0	0	0	0	0	0	0.0
Tea, instant, sweetened with sodium saccharin, lemon-flavored, prepared								
1 fl oz (30g)	1	0	0	0	0	0	3	0.0
Tea, instant, sweetened with sugar, lemon-flavored, with added ascorbic acid, powder, prepared								
1 cup (8 fl oz) (259g)	88	0	0	21	0	0	8	0.0
Tea, instant, sweetened with sugar, lemon-flavored, without added ascorbic acid, powder, prepared								
1 cup (8 fl oz) (259g)	88	0	0	21	0	0	8	0.0
Tea, instant, sweetened with sugar, lemon-flavored, without added ascorbic acid, powder								
1 serving (3 heaping teaspoons) (23g)	89	0	0	23	0	0	1	0.0
Tea, instant, unsweetened, lemon-flavored, powder, prepared								
1 cup (8 fl oz) (238g)	5	0	0	0	0	0	14	0.0
Tea, instant, unsweetened, powder, prepared								
1 fl oz (30g)	0	0	0	0	0	0	1	0.0
Thirst quencher drink, bottled								
1 fl oz (30g)	8	0	0	2	0	0	12	0.0
Water, bottled, PERRIER								
1 fl oz (30g)	0	0	0	0	0	0	0	0.0

Snacks and Sweets

Food Serving size	Cal.	Fat cal.	Prot.	Carb.	Fat	Chol.	Sod.	Fiber
Candies								
Baking chocolate, Mexican, squares 1 tablet (20g)	85	27	1	15	3	0	1	0.8
Baking chocolate, unsweetened, liquid 1 oz (28g)	132	113	3	10	13	0	3	3.6
Baking chocolate, unsweetened, squares 1 square (1 oz) (28g)	146	129	3	8	15	0	4	4.2
Candies, butterscotch 1 piece (6g)	24	0	0	6	0	1	3	0.0
Candies, caramels, chocolate-flavor roll 1 piece (7g)	25	1	0	6	0	0	2	0.1
Candies, caramels 1 piece (10g)	38	7	1	8	1	1	25	0.1
Candies, carob 1 oz (28g)	151	78	2	16	9	1	30	1.1
Candies, butterscotch, confectioner's coating 1 oz (28g)	146	70	1	19	8	0	26	0.0
Candies, peanut butter, confectioner's coating 1 oz (28g)	139	71	5	13	8	0	70	0.3
Candies, yogurt, confectioner's coating 100 grams	521	243	6	64	27	1	90	0.0
Candies, divinity, prepared-from-recipe 1 piece (11g)	38	0	0	10	0	0	5	0.0

Food Serving size	Cal.	Fat cal.	Prot.	Carb.	Fat	Chol.	Sod.	Fiber
Candies, fondant, prepared-from-recipe								
1 piece (16g)	57	0	0	15	0	0	6	0.0
Candies, fudge, brown sugar, with nuts, prepared-from-recipe								
1 piece (14g)	55	0	0	11	1	1	14	0.1
Candies, fudge, chocolate marshmallow, prepared-from-recipe								
1 piece (20g)	84	0	0	14	3	5	21	0.0
Candies, fudge, chocolate marshmallow, with nuts, prepared-from-recipe								
1 piece (22g)	96	0	1	15	4	5	21	0.4
Candies, fudge, chocolate, prepared-from-recipe								
1 piece (17g)	65	0	0	14	1	2	11	0.2
Candies, fudge, chocolate, with nuts, prepared-from-recipe								
1 piece (19g)	81	0	1	14	3	3	11	0.2
Candies, fudge, peanut butter, prepared-from-recipe								
1 piece (16g)	59	0	1	12	1	1	12	0.2
Candies, fudge, vanilla, prepared-from-recipe								
1 piece (16g)	59	0	0	13	1	3	11	0.0
Candies, fudge, vanilla, with nuts, prepared-from-recipe								
1 piece (15g)	62	0	0	11	2	2	9	0.2
Candies, gumdrops, starch jelly pieces								
10 gumdrops (36g)	139	0	0	36	0	0	16	0.0
Candies, halvah, plain								
100 grams	469	187	12	60	22	0	195	4.0
Candies, hard								
1 piece (6g)	22	0	0	6	0	0	2	0.0
Candies, jellybeans								
10 small (11g)	40	0	0	10	0	0	3	0.0
Candies, marshmallows								
10 miniatures (7g)	22	0	0	6	0	0	3	0.0
Candies, milk chocolate coated peanuts								
10 pieces (40g)	208	117	5	20	14	4	16	1.6
Candies, milk chocolate coated raisins								
10 pieces (10g)	39	13	0	7	2	0	4	0.4

Food Serving size	Cal.	Fat cal.	Prot.	Carb.	Fat	Chol.	Sod.	Fiber
Candies, milk chocolate, with almonds								
1 bar (1.45 oz) (41g)	216	120	4	22	14	8	30	2.5
Candies, milk chocolate, with rice cereal								
1 bar (1.4 oz) (40g)	198	90	2	25	10	8	58	1.2
Candies, milk chocolate								
1 miniature bar (7g)	36	19	0	4	2	2	6	0.2
Candies, peanut bar								
1 oz (28g)	146	80	4	13	10	2	67	0.8
Candies, peanut brittle, prepared-from-recipe								
1 oz (28g)	127	0	2	19	5	4	127	0.6
Candies, praline, prepared-from-recipe								
1 piece (39g)	177	0	1	24	9	0	24	1.2
Candies, semisweet chocolate, made with butter 1 cup (6 oz package)								
chips (170g)	811	434	7	107	51	31	19	10.2
Candies, semisweet chocolate 1 cup (6 oz package)								
chips (168g)	805	428	7	106	50	0	18	10.1
Candies, sesame crunch								
1 piece (2g)	10	6	0	1	1	0	0	0.2
Candies, sweet chocolate coated fondant								
1 small patty (11g)	40	8	0	9	1	0	3	0.1
Candies, sweet chocolate								
1 oz (28g)	141	82	1	17	10	0	4	1.7
Candies, taffy, prepared-from-recipe								
1 piece (15g)	56	0	0	14	0	1	13	0.0
Candies, toffee, prepared-from-recipe								
1 piece (12g)	65	0	0	8	4	13	22	0.0
Candies, truffles, prepared-from-recipe								
1 piece (12g)	59	0	1	5	4	6	9	0.2
Chewing gum								
1 stick (3g)	10	0	0	3	0	0	0	0.0
Sweets, confectioner's coating, white								
1 bar (3 oz) (85g)	458	239	5	50	27	18	77	0.0

Food Serving size	Cal.	Fat cal.	Prot.	Carb.	Fat	Chol.	Sod.	Fiber

Chips and Pretzels

Banana chips
1 oz (28g)

	145	82	1	16	10	0	2	2.2

Corn-based snacks, extruded, chips, barbecue-flavor
1 oz (28g)

	146	80	2	16	9	0	214	1.4

Corn-based snacks, extruded, chips, plain
1 oz (28g)

	151	81	2	16	9	0	176	1.4

Corn-based snacks, extruded, cones, nacho-flavor
1 oz (28g)

	150	77	2	16	9	1	267	0.3

Corn-based snacks, extruded, cones, plain
1 oz (28g)

	143	65	2	18	8	0	286	0.3

Corn-based snacks, extruded, onion-flavor
1 oz (28g)

	140	57	2	18	6	0	275	1.1

Corn-based snacks, extruded, puffs or twists, cheese-flavor, enriched
1 oz (28g)

	155	84	2	15	10	1	294	0.3

Corn-based snacks, extruded, puffs or twists, cheese-flavor
1 oz (28g)

	155	84	2	15	10	1	294	0.3

Cornnuts, barbecue-flavor
1 oz (28g)

	122	34	3	20	4	0	273	2.2

Cornnuts, nacho-flavor
1 oz (28g)

	123	34	3	20	4	1	178	2.2

Cornnuts, plain
1 oz (28g)

	123	34	2	20	4	0	154	2.0

Pork skins, barbecue-flavor
$\frac{1}{2}$ oz (14g)

	75	40	8	0	4	16	373	

Pork skins, plain
$\frac{1}{2}$ oz (14g)

	76	39	9	0	4	13	257	0.0

Potato chips, barbecue-flavor
1 oz (28g)

	137	78	2	15	9	0	210	1.1

Potato chips, cheese-flavor
1 oz (28g)

	139	67	2	16	8	1	222	1.4

Potato chips, light
1 oz (28g)

	132	52	2	19	6	0	138	1.7

Food Serving size	Cal.	Fat cal.	Prot.	Carb.	Fat	Chol.	Sod.	Fiber
Potato chips, made from dried potatoes, cheese-flavor								
1 oz (28g)	154	91	2	14	10	1	211	0.8
Potato chips, made from dried potatoes, light								
1 oz (28g)	140	64	2	18	7	0	120	1.1
Potato chips, made from dried potatoes, plain								
1 oz (28g)	156	94	2	14	11	0	184	1.1
Potato chips, made from dried potatoes, sour-cream and onion-flavor								
1 oz (28g)	153	91	2	14	10	1	202	0.3
Potato chips, plain, made with partially hydrogenated soybean oil, salted								
1 oz (28g)	150	86	2	15	10	0	166	1.4
Potato chips, plain, made with partially hydrogenated soybean oil, unsalted								
1 oz (28g)	150	86	2	15	10	0	2	1.4
Potato chips, plain, salted								
1 oz (28g)	150	86	2	15	10	0	166	1.1
Potato chips, plain, unsalted								
1 oz (28g)	150	86	2	15	10	0	2	1.4
Potato chips, sour-cream-and-onion-flavor								
1 oz (28g)	149	84	2	15	10	2	175	1.4
Potato sticks								
½ cup (18g)	94	51	1	10	6	0	45	0.5
Pretzels, hard, confectioner's coating, chocolate-flavor								
1 pretzel (11g)	50	16	1	8	2	0	63	
Pretzels, hard, plain, made with unenriched flour, salted								
1 oz (28g)	107	10	3	22	1	0	480	0.8
Pretzels, hard, plain, made with unenriched flour, unsalted								
1 oz (28g)	107	10	3	22	1	0	81	0.8
Pretzels, hard, plain, salted								
1 oz (28g)	107	10	3	22	1	0	480	0.8
Pretzels, hard, plain, unsalted								
1 oz (28g)	107	10	3	22	1	0	81	0.8
Pretzels, hard, whole-wheat								
1 oz (28g)	101	7	3	23	1	0	57	2.2

Food Serving size	Cal.	Fat cal.	Prot.	Carb.	Fat	Chol.	Sod.	Fiber
Taro chips 10 chips (23g)	115	51	0	16	6	0	79	1.6
Tortilla chips, nacho-flavor, light 1 oz (28g)	125	37	3	20	4	1	281	1.4
Tortilla chips, nacho-flavor 1 oz (28g)	139	64	2	17	7	1	198	1.4
Tortilla chips, plain 1 oz (28g)	140	64	2	18	7	0	148	1.7
Tortilla chips, ranch-flavor 1 oz (28g)	137	59	2	18	7	0	171	1.1
Tortilla chips, taco-flavor 1 oz (28g)	134	58	2	18	7	1	220	1.4

Desserts

Food Serving size	Cal.	Fat cal.	Prot.	Carb.	Fat	Chol.	Sod.	Fiber
Desserts, apple crisp, prepared-from-recipe $\frac{1}{2}$ cup (141g)	230	0	3	45	6	0	257	2.8
Desserts, bread pudding, prepared-from-recipe $\frac{1}{2}$ cup (126g)	212	0	6	32	8	83	291	1.3
Desserts, egg custards, baked, prepared-from-recipe $\frac{1}{2}$ cup (141g)	148	0	7	16	7	123	109	0.0
Desserts, egg custards, dry mix, prepared with 2% milk $\frac{1}{2}$ cup (133g)	149	0	5	24	4	74	200	0.0
Desserts, egg custards, dry mix, prepared with whole milk $\frac{1}{2}$ cup (133g)	162	0	5	24	5	81	198	0.0
Desserts, egg custards, dry mix amount to make $\frac{1}{2}$ cup (21g)	86	11	1	17	1	63	136	0.0
Desserts, flan, caramel custard, dry mix, prepared with 2% milk $\frac{1}{2}$ cup (133g)	136	0	4	25	3	9	67	0.0
Desserts, flan, caramel custard, dry mix, prepared with whole milk $\frac{1}{2}$ cup (133g)	150	0	4	25	4	16	65	0.0
Desserts, flan, caramel custard, prepared-from-recipe $\frac{1}{2}$ cup (153g)	220	0	6	35	6	141	86	0.0

Food Serving size	Cal.	Fat cal.	Prot.	Carb.	Fat	Chol.	Sod.	Fiber
Desserts, gelatins, dry mix, prepared with water								
½ cup (135g)	80	0	1	19	0	0	57	0.0
Desserts, gelatins, dry mix, reduced calorie, with aspartame, prepared with water								
½ cup (117g)	8	0	1	1	0	0	56	0.0
Desserts, gelatins, dry mix, reduced calorie, with aspartame								
1 tablespoon (9g)	31	0	5	3	0	0	195	0.0
Desserts, gelatins, dry mix, with fruit, prepared-from-recipe								
½ cup (106g)	73	0	1	18	0	0	30	1.1
Desserts, mousse, chocolate, prepared-from-recipe								
½ cup (202g)	446	0	8	32	32	299	87	2.0
Desserts, puddings, banana, dry mix, instant, prepared with 2% milk								
½ cup (147g)	153	0	4	29	3	9	435	0.0
Desserts, puddings, banana, dry mix, instant, prepared with whole milk								
½ cup (147g)	166	0	4	29	4	16	434	0.0
Desserts, puddings, banana, dry mix, regular, prepared with 2% milk								
½ cup (140g)	143	0	4	25	3	10	232	0.0
Desserts, puddings, banana, dry mix, regular, prepared with whole milk								
½ cup (140g)	157	0	4	25	4	17	231	0.0
Desserts, puddings, banana, ready-to-eat								
1 oz (28g)	36	10	1	6	1	0	55	0.0
Desserts, puddings, chocolate, dry mix, instant, prepared with 2% milk								
½ cup (147g)	150	0	4	28	3	9	417	0.0
Desserts, puddings, chocolate, dry mix, instant, prepared with whole milk								
½ cup (147g)	163	0	4	28	4	16	417	1.5
Desserts, puddings, chocolate, dry mix, regular, prepared with 2% milk								
½ cup (142g)	151	0	4	28	3	10	149	0.0
Desserts, puddings, chocolate, dry mix, regular, prepared with whole milk								
½ cup (142g)	158	0	4	26	4	17	146	1.4

Food Serving size	Cal.	Fat cal.	Prot.	Carb.	Fat	Chol.	Sod.	Fiber
Desserts, puddings, chocolate, prepared-from-recipe, prepared with 2% milk								
$\frac{1}{2}$ cup (157g)	206	0	5	41	3	9	138	1.6
Desserts, puddings, chocolate, prepared-from-recipe, prepared with whole milk								
$\frac{1}{2}$ cup (157g)	221	0	5	41	6	17	137	1.6
Desserts, puddings, chocolate, ready-to-eat								
1 oz (28g)	37	10	1	6	1	1	36	0.3
Desserts, puddings, coconut cream, dry mix, instant, prepared with 2% milk								
$\frac{1}{2}$ cup (147g)	157	0	4	28	3	9	362	0.0
Desserts, puddings, coconut cream, dry mix, instant, prepared with whole milk								
$\frac{1}{2}$ cup (147g)	172	0	4	28	6	16	362	0.0
Desserts, puddings, coconut cream, dry mix, regular, prepared with 2% milk								
$\frac{1}{2}$ cup (140g)	146	0	4	25	3	10	228	0.0
Desserts, puddings, coconut cream, dry mix, regular, prepared with whole milk								
$\frac{1}{2}$ cup (140g)	160	0	4	25	6	17	227	0.0
Desserts, puddings, lemon, dry mix, instant, prepared with 2% milk								
$\frac{1}{2}$ cup (147g)	154	0	4	29	3	9	394	0.0
Desserts, puddings, lemon, dry mix, instant, prepared with whole milk								
$\frac{1}{2}$ cup (147g)	169	0	4	29	4	16	392	0.0
Desserts, puddings, lemon, dry mix, regular, prepared with sugar, egg yolk and water								
$\frac{1}{2}$ cup (146g)	164	0	1	37	1	77	93	0.0
Desserts, puddings, lemon, ready-to-eat								
1 oz (28g)	35	7	0	7	1	0	39	0.0
Desserts, puddings, rice, dry mix, prepared with 2% milk								
$\frac{1}{2}$ cup (144g)	161	0	4	30	3	9	158	0.0
Desserts, puddings, rice, dry mix, prepared with whole milk								
$\frac{1}{2}$ cup (144g)	176	0	4	30	4	16	157	0.0
Desserts, puddings, rice, prepared-from-recipe								
$\frac{1}{2}$ cup (152g)	217	0	6	40	5	17	85	0.0

Food Serving size	Cal.	Fat cal.	Prot.	Carb.	Fat	Chol.	Sod.	Fiber
Desserts, puddings, rice, ready-to-eat								
1 oz (28g)	46	20	1	6	2	0	24	0.0
Desserts, puddings, tapioca, dry mix, prepared with 2% milk								
½ cup (141g)	147	0	4	28	3	8	172	0.0
Desserts, puddings, tapioca, dry mix, prepared with whole milk								
½ cup (141g)	161	0	4	28	4	17	171	0.0
Desserts, puddings, tapioca, prepared-from-recipe								
½ cup (152g)	190	0	8	26	6	125	289	0.0
Desserts, puddings, tapioca, ready-to-eat								
1 oz (28g)	33	10	1	5	1	0	33	0.0
Desserts, puddings, vanilla, dry mix, instant, prepared with 2% milk								
½ cup (142g)	148	0	4	28	3	9	406	0.0
Desserts, puddings, vanilla, dry mix, instant, prepared with whole milk								
½ cup (142g)	162	0	4	28	4	16	406	0.0
Desserts, puddings, vanilla, dry mix, regular, prepared with 2% milk								
½ cup (140g)	141	0	4	27	3	10	224	0.0
Desserts, puddings, vanilla, dry mix, regular, prepared with whole milk								
½ cup (140g)	155	0	4	25	4	17	224	0.0
Desserts, puddings, vanilla, prepared-from-recipe								
½ cup (123g)	130	0	4	20	4	16	113	0.0
Desserts, puddings, vanilla, ready-to-eat								
1 oz (28g)	36	10	1	6	1	2	38	0.0
Desserts, rennin, chocolate, dry mix, prepared with 2% milk								
½ cup (136g)	110	0	4	19	3	10	71	0.0
Desserts, rennin, chocolate, dry mix, prepared with whole milk								
½ cup (136g)	125	0	4	18	4	16	69	0.0
Desserts, rennin, vanilla, dry mix, prepared with 2% milk								
½ cup (133g)	101	0	4	16	3	9	61	0.0
Desserts, rennin, vanilla, dry mix, prepared with whole milk								
½ cup (133g)	116	0	4	16	4	17	61	0.0
Desserts, rennin, vanilla, prepared-from-recipe								
½ cup (137g)	112	0	4	15	4	16	96	0.0

Food Serving size	Cal.	Fat cal.	Prot.	Carb.	Fat	Chol.	Sod.	Fiber

Frostings and Fillings

Frostings, chocolate, creamy, dry mix, prepared with butter
| $\frac{1}{12}$ package (42g) | 160 | 0 | 0 | 30 | 5 | 10 | 63 | 0.8 |

Frostings, chocolate, creamy, dry mix, prepared with margarine
| $\frac{1}{12}$ package (42g) | 161 | 0 | 0 | 30 | 5 | 0 | 69 | 0.8 |

Frostings, chocolate, creamy, prepared-from-recipe with butter
| $\frac{1}{12}$ package (50g) | 200 | 0 | 1 | 39 | 6 | 15 | 95 | 1.0 |

Frostings, chocolate, creamy, prepared-from-recipe with margarine
| $\frac{1}{12}$ package (50g) | 201 | 0 | 1 | 39 | 6 | 1 | 103 | 1.0 |

Frostings, chocolate, creamy, ready-to-eat, without added phosphorus, vitamin A
| $\frac{1}{12}$ package (38g) | 151 | 60 | 0 | 24 | 7 | 0 | 70 | 0.4 |

Frostings, chocolate, creamy, ready-to-eat
| $\frac{1}{12}$ package (38g) | 151 | 60 | 0 | 24 | 7 | 0 | 70 | 0.4 |

Frostings, coconut-nut, ready-to-eat, without added phosphorus
| $\frac{1}{12}$ package (38g) | 157 | 78 | 1 | 20 | 9 | 0 | 74 | 0.4 |

Frostings, coconut-nut, ready-to-eat
| $\frac{1}{12}$ package (38g) | 157 | 78 | 1 | 20 | 9 | 0 | 74 | 0.4 |

Frostings, cream cheese flavor, ready-to-eat, without added sodium, vitamin A
| $\frac{1}{12}$ package (38g) | 157 | 57 | 0 | 25 | 6 | 0 | 15 | 0.0 |

Frostings, cream cheese flavor, ready-to-eat
| $\frac{1}{12}$ package (38g) | 157 | 57 | 0 | 25 | 6 | 0 | 90 | 0.0 |

Frostings, glaze, prepared-from-recipe
| recipe yield (327g) | 1174 | 0 | 3 | 242 | 26 | 7 | 307 | 0.0 |

Frostings, seven minute, prepared-from-recipe
| recipe yield (387g) | 1231 | 0 | 8 | 310 | 0 | 0 | 658 | 0.0 |

Frostings, sour cream flavor, ready-to-eat, without added phosphorus, potassium
| $\frac{1}{12}$ package (38g) | 157 | 56 | 0 | 26 | 6 | 0 | 78 | 0.0 |

Frostings, sour cream flavor, ready-to-eat
| $\frac{1}{12}$ package (38g) | 157 | 56 | 0 | 26 | 6 | 0 | 78 | 0.0 |

Food Serving size	Cal.	Fat cal.	Prot.	Carb.	Fat	Chol.	Sod.	Fiber
Frostings, vanilla, creamy, dry mix, prepared with butter								
$\frac{1}{12}$ package (43g)	182	0	0	31	7	10	90	0.0
Frostings, vanilla, creamy, dry mix, prepared with margarine								
$\frac{1}{12}$ package (43g)	182	0	0	31	7	0	95	0.0
Frostings, vanilla, creamy, prepared-from-recipe with butter								
recipe yield (574g)	1969	0	6	448	23	69	367	0.0
Frostings, vanilla, creamy, prepared-from-recipe with margarine								
recipe yield (574g)	2325	0	0	453	63	6	1177	0.0
Frostings, vanilla, creamy, ready-to-eat, without added phosphorus, vitamin A								
$\frac{1}{12}$ package (38g)	159	57	0	26	6	0	34	0.0
Frostings, vanilla, creamy, ready-to-eat								
$\frac{1}{12}$ package (38g)	159	57	0	26	6	0	34	0.0
Frostings, white, fluffy, dry mix, prepared with water								
$\frac{1}{12}$ package (26g)	63	0	1	16	0	0	41	0.0
Pie fillings, canned, apple								
$\frac{1}{8}$ can (74g)	75	0	0	19	0	0	33	0.7
Pie fillings, canned, cherry								
$\frac{1}{8}$ can (74g)	85	0	0	21	0	0	7	0.7

Frozen Desserts

Food Serving size	Cal.	Fat cal.	Prot.	Carb.	Fat	Chol.	Sod.	Fiber
Frozen desserts, fruit and juice bars								
1 bar (2.5 fl oz) (77g)	63	0	1	15	0	0	3	0.0
Frozen desserts, ice cream, chocolate								
1 individual cup								
(3.5 fl oz) (58g)	125	56	2	16	6	20	44	0.6
Frozen desserts, ice cream, French vanilla, soft-serve								
$\frac{1}{2}$ cup (4 fl oz) (86g)	185	98	3	19	11	78	52	0.0
Frozen desserts, ice cream, strawberry								
1 individual cup								
(3.5 fl oz) (58g)	111	41	2	16	5	17	35	0.0
Frozen desserts, ice cream, vanilla, rich								
$\frac{1}{2}$ cup (4 fl oz) (74g)	178	104	3	16	12	45	41	0.0
Frozen desserts, ice cream, vanilla								
1 individual cup								
(3.5 fl oz) (58g)	117	56	2	14	6	26	46	0.0

Food Serving size	Cal.	Fat cal.	Prot.	Carb.	Fat	Chol.	Sod.	Fiber
Frozen desserts, ice milk, vanilla, soft serve								
$\frac{1}{2}$ cup (4 fl oz) (88g)	111	23	4	19	3	11	62	0.0
Frozen desserts, ice milk, vanilla 1 individual cup								
(3.5 fl oz) (65g)	90	23	3	15	3	9	55	0.0
Frozen desserts, ice pops, with added ascorbic acid								
1 bar (1.75 fl oz) (52g)	37	0	0	10	0	0	6	0.0
Frozen desserts, ice pops								
1 bar (1.75 fl oz) (52g)	37	0	0	10	0	0	6	0.0
Frozen desserts, ice, Italian, restaurant-prepared								
1 fl oz (29g)	15	0	0	4	0	0	1	0.0
Frozen desserts, ices, water, fruit, reduced calorie, with aspartame								
1 bar (51g)	12	0	0	3	0	0	3	0.0
Frozen desserts, ices, water, lime								
$\frac{1}{2}$ cup (4 fl oz) (99g)	127	0	0	33	0	0	22	0.0
Frozen desserts, ices, water, pineapple-coconut								
$\frac{1}{2}$ cup (4 fl oz) (99g)	112	25	0	24	3	0	35	1.0
Frozen desserts, sherbet, orange								
1 bar (2.75 fl oz) (66g)	91	12	1	20	1	3	30	0.0
Frozen desserts, yogurt, chocolate, soft-serve								
$\frac{1}{2}$ cup (4 fl oz) (72g)	115	38	3	18	4	4	71	1.4
Frozen desserts, yogurt, vanilla, soft-serve								
$\frac{1}{2}$ cup (72g)	114	38	3	17	4	1	63	0.0

Fruit Snacks

Food Serving size	Cal.	Fat cal.	Prot.	Carb.	Fat	Chol.	Sod.	Fiber
Fruit butters, apple								
1 tablespoon (18g)	33	0	0	9	0	0	0	0.2
Fruit leather, bars, with cream								
1 bar (24g)	89	17	0	19	2	1	23	1.0
Fruit leather, bars								
1 bar (23g)	81	10	0	18	1	0	18	0.9
Fruit leather, pieces								
1 package (27g)	92	17	0	21	2	0	109	1.1
Fruit leather, rolls								
1 small (14g)	49	4	0	12	0	0	9	0.6

Food Serving size	Cal.	Fat cal.	Prot.	Carb.	Fat	Chol.	Sod.	Fiber

Granola Bars and Trail Mixes

Granola bars, hard, almond
| 1 bar (24g) | 119 | 54 | 2 | 15 | 6 | 0 | 61 | 1.2 |

Granola bars, hard, chocolate chip
| 1 bar (24g) | 105 | 33 | 2 | 17 | 4 | 0 | 83 | 1.0 |

Granola bars, hard, peanut butter
| 1 bar (24g) | 116 | 50 | 2 | 15 | 6 | 0 | 68 | 0.7 |

Granola bars, hard, peanut
| 1 oz (28g) | 134 | 51 | 3 | 18 | 6 | 0 | 78 | 1.1 |

Granola bars, hard, plain
| 1 bar (24g) | 113 | 42 | 2 | 15 | 5 | 0 | 71 | 1.2 |

Granola bars, soft, coated, milk chocolate coating, chocolate chip
| 1 bar (1 oz) (28g) | 130 | 60 | 2 | 18 | 7 | 1 | 56 | 0.8 |

Granola bars, soft, coated, milk chocolate coating, peanut butter
| 1 oz (28g) | 143 | 75 | 3 | 15 | 9 | 3 | 54 | 0.8 |

Granola bars, soft, uncoated, chocolate chip, graham and marshmallow
| 1 bar (1 oz) (28g) | 120 | 38 | 2 | 20 | 4 | 0 | 88 | 1.1 |

Granola bars, soft, uncoated, chocolate chip
| 1 bar (1 oz) (28g) | 118 | 40 | 2 | 19 | 5 | 0 | 76 | 1.4 |

Granola bars, soft, uncoated, nut and raisin
| 1 bar (1 oz) (28g) | 127 | 47 | 2 | 18 | 6 | 0 | 71 | 1.7 |

Granola bars, soft, uncoated, peanut butter and chocolate chip
| 1 bar (1 oz) (28g) | 121 | 47 | 3 | 17 | 6 | 0 | 92 | 1.1 |

Granola bars, soft, uncoated, peanut butter
| 1 bar (1 oz) (28g) | 119 | 38 | 3 | 18 | 4 | 0 | 115 | 1.1 |

Granola bars, soft, uncoated, plain
| 1 bar (1 oz) (28g) | 124 | 41 | 2 | 19 | 5 | 0 | 78 | 1.4 |

Granola bars, soft, uncoated, raisin
| 1 bar (1 oz) (28g) | 125 | 42 | 2 | 18 | 5 | 0 | 79 | 1.1 |

Trail mix, regular, unsalted
| 1 oz (28g) | 129 | 68 | 4 | 13 | 8 | 0 | 3 | |

Food Serving size	Cal.	Fat cal.	Prot.	Carb.	Fat	Chol.	Sod.	Fiber
Trail mix, regular, with chocolate chips, salted nuts and seeds								
1 oz (28g)	136	75	4	13	9	1	34	
Trail mix, regular, with chocolate chips, unsalted nuts and seeds								
1 oz (28g)	136	75	4	13	9	1	8	
Trail mix, regular								
1 oz (28g)	129	68	4	13	8	0	64	
Trail mix, tropical								
1 oz (28g)	114	0	2	18	5	0	3	

Popcorn

Food Serving size	Cal.	Fat cal.	Prot.	Carb.	Fat	Chol.	Sod.	Fiber
Popcorn, air-popped, white popcorn								
1 cup (8g)	31	3	1	6	0	0	0	1.2
Popcorn, air-popped								
1 cup (8g)	31	3	1	6	0	0	0	1.2
Popcorn, cakes								
1 cake (10g)	38	3	1	8	0	0	29	0.3
Popcorn, caramel-coated, with peanuts								
1 oz (approx $\frac{2}{3}$ cup) (28g)	112	19	2	23	2	0	83	1.1
Popcorn, caramel-coated, without peanuts								
1 oz (28g)	121	32	1	22	4	1	58	1.4
Popcorn, cheese-flavor								
1 cup (11g)	58	32	1	6	4	1	98	1.1
Popcorn, oil-popped, white popcorn								
1 cup (11g)	55	27	1	6	3	0	97	1.1
Popcorn, oil-popped								
1 cup (11g)	55	27	1	6	3	0	97	1.1

Rice Cakes

Food Serving size	Cal.	Fat cal.	Prot.	Carb.	Fat	Chol.	Sod.	Fiber
Rice cakes, brown rice, buckwheat, unsalted								
1 cake (9g)	34	3	1	7	0	0	0	
Rice cakes, brown rice, buckwheat								
1 cake (9g)	34	3	1	7	0	0	10	0.4

Food Serving size	Cal.	Fat cal.	Prot.	Carb.	Fat	Chol.	Sod.	Fiber
Rice cakes, brown rice, corn 1 cake (9g)	35	2	1	7	0	0	26	0.3
Rice cakes, brown rice, multigrain, unsalted 1 cake (9g)	35	3	1	7	0	0	0	
Rice cakes, brown rice, multigrain 1 cake (9g)	35	3	1	7	0	0	23	0.3
Rice cakes, brown rice, plain, unsalted 1 cake (9g)	35	2	1	7	0	0	2	0.4
Rice cakes, brown rice, plain 1 cake (9g)	35	2	1	7	0	0	29	0.4
Rice cakes, brown rice, rye 1 cake (9g)	35	3	1	7	0	0	10	0.4
Rice cakes, brown rice, sesame seed, unsalted 1 cake (9g)	35	3	1	7	0	0	0	
Rice cakes, brown rice, sesame seed 1 cake (9g)	35	3	1	7	0	0	20	0.4

Sugars, Syrups, and Toppings

Food Serving size	Cal.	Fat cal.	Prot.	Carb.	Fat	Chol.	Sod.	Fiber
Honey, strained or extracted 1 tablespoon (21g)	64	0	0	17	0	0	1	0.0
Molasses, blackstrap 1 tablespoon (20g)	47	0	0	12	0	0	11	0.0
Molasses 1 tablespoon (20g)	53	0	0	14	0	0	7	0.0
Sugars, brown 1 cup, unpacked (145g)	545	0	0	141	0	0	57	0.0
Sugars, granulated 1 teaspoon (4g)	15	0	0	4	0	0	0	0.0
Sugars, maple 1 teaspoon (3g)	11	0	0	3	0	0	0	0.0
Sugars, powdered 1 tablespoon, unsifted (8g)	31	0	0	8	0	0	0	0.0
Syrups, chocolate, fudge-type 1 tablespoon (21g)	73	24	1	12	3	3	27	0.2

Food Serving size	Cal.	Fat cal.	Prot.	Carb.	Fat	Chol.	Sod.	Fiber
Syrups, corn, dark 1 tablespoon (20g)	56	0	0	15	0	0	31	0.0
Syrups, corn, high-fructose 1 tablespoon (19g)	53	0	0	14	0	0	0	0.0
Syrups, corn, light 1 tablespoon (20g)	56	0	0	15	0	0	24	0.0
Syrups, malt 1 tablespoon (24g)	76	0	1	17	0	0	8	0.0
Syrups, maple 1 tablespoon (20g)	52	0	0	13	0	0	2	0.0
Syrups, sorghum 1 tablespoon (21g)	61	0	0	16	0	0	2	0.0
Syrups, table blends, cane and 15% maple 1 tablespoon (20g)	56	0	0	15	0	0	21	0.0
Syrups, table blends, corn, refiner, and sugar 1 tablespoon (20g)	64	0	0	17	0	0	14	0.0
Syrups, table blends, pancake, reduced-calorie 1 tablespoon (15g)	25	0	0	7	0	0	30	0.0
Syrups, table blends, pancake, with 2% maple, with added potassium 1 tablespoon (20g)	53	0	0	14	0	0	12	0.0
Syrups, table blends, pancake, with 2% maple 1 tablespoon (20g)	53	0	0	14	0	0	12	0.0
Syrups, table blends, pancake, with butter 1 tablespoon (20g)	59	0	0	15	0	1	20	0.0
Syrups, table blends, pancake 1 tablespoon (20g)	57	0	0	15	0	0	17	0.0
Toppings, butterscotch or caramel 2 tablespoons (41g)	103	0	1	27	0	0	143	0.4
Toppings, marshmallow cream 1 oz (28g)	87	0	1	22	0	0	13	0.0
Toppings, nuts in syrup 2 tablespoons (41g)	167	75	2	22	9	0	17	0.8
Toppings, pineapple 2 tablespoons (42g)	106	0	0	28	0	0	26	0.4

Food Serving size	Cal.	Fat cal.	Prot.	Carb.	Fat	Chol.	Sod.	Fiber
Toppings, strawberry 2 tablespoons (42g)	107	0	0	28	0	0	9	0.4

Miscellaneous Snacks

Food Serving size	Cal.	Fat cal.	Prot.	Carb.	Fat	Chol.	Sod.	Fiber
Beef jerky, chopped and formed 1 large piece (20g)	82		7	2	5	10	443	0.4
Cocoa, dry powder, unsweetened 1 tablespoon (5g)	11	6	1	3	1	0	1	1.6
Corn cakes, very low sodium 1 cake (9g)	35	2	1	7	0	0	3	
Corn cakes 1 cake (9g)	35	2	1	7	0	0	44	0.2
Crisped rice bar, chocolate chip 1 bar (1 oz) (28g)	113	34	1	20	4	0	78	0.6
Jams and preserves, apricot 1 packet (0.5 oz) (14g)	34	0	0	9	0	0	6	0.1
Jams and preserves 1 packet (0.5 oz) (14g)	34	0	0	9	0	0	6	0.1
Jellies 1 tablespoon (19g)	51	0	0	13	0	0	7	0.2
Marmalade, orange 1 tablespoon (20g)	49	0	0	13	0	0	11	0.0
Meat-based sticks, smoked 1 stick (20g)	110	90	4	1	10	27	296	
Oriental mix, rice-based 1 oz (28g)	154	0	5	15	7	0	116	3.6
Sesame sticks, wheat-based, salted 1 oz (28g)	151	90	3	13	10	0	417	0.8
Sesame sticks, wheat-based, unsalted 1 oz (28g)	151	90	3	13	10	0	8	

Processed Foods

Food Serving size	Cal.	Fat cal.	Prot.	Carb.	Fat	Chol.	Sod.	Fiber
Beef macaroni, frozen entree 1 serving (240g)	211	22	14	34	2	14	444	4.8
Beef stew 1 cup (252g)	192	45	15	20	5	33	1187	2.5
Biscuit with egg and sausage 1 biscuit (180g)	581	348	20	41	40	302	1141	0.0
Biscuit with egg and steak 1 biscuit (148g)	410	248	18	21	28	272	888	
Biscuit, with egg and bacon 1 biscuit (150g)	458	277	17	29	32	353	999	0.0
Biscuit, with egg and ham 1 biscuit (192g)	442	237	21	31	27	300	1382	0.0
Biscuit, with egg, cheese, and bacon 1 biscuit (144g)	477	279	16	33	32	261	1260	
Biscuit, with egg 1 biscuit (136g)	316	176	11	24	20	233	654	
Biscuit, with ham 1 biscuit (113g)	386	157	14	44	18	25	1433	1.1
Biscuit, with sausage 1 biscuit (124g)	485	282	12	40	32	35	1071	1.2
Biscuit, with steak 1 biscuit (141g)	455	222	13	44	25	25	795	
Breakfast patties 1 patty (38g)	79	24	10	4	3	1	259	1.9

Food Serving size	Cal.	Fat cal.	Prot.	Carb.	Fat	Chol.	Sod.	Fiber
Brownie 1 brownie (2″ square) (60g)	243	89	3	39	10	10	153	
Burrito, with beans and cheese 2 pieces (186g)	378	97	15	56	11	28	1166	
Burrito, with beans and chili peppers 2 pieces (204g)	412	120	16	57	14	33	1044	
Burrito, with beans and meat 2 pieces (231g)	508	161	23	67	18	49	1335	
Burrito, with beans, cheese, and beef 2 pieces (203g)	331	124	14	41	14	124	991	
Burrito, with beans, cheese, and chili peppers 2 pieces (336g)	662	203	34	84	24	158	2060	
Burrito, with beans 2 pieces (217g)	447	109	13	72	13	4	985	
Burrito, with beef and chili peppers 2 pieces (201g)	426	141	22	50	16	54	1116	
Burrito, with beef, cheese, and chili peppers 2 pieces (304g)	632	213	40	64	24	170	2092	
Burrito, with beef 2 pieces (220g)	524	173	26	59	20	64	1492	
Burrito, with fruit (apple or cherry) 1 small burrito (74g)	231	86	2	35	10	4	212	
Cheeseburger, large, double patty, with condiments and vegetables 1 sandwich (258g)	704	391	39	39	44	142	1148	
Cheeseburger, large, single meat patty, plain 1 sandwich (185g)	609	297	30	48	33	96	1589	
Cheeseburger, large, single meat patty, with bacon and condiments 1 sandwich (195g)	608	330	31	37	37	111	1043	
Cheeseburger, large, single patty, with condiments and vegetables 1 sandwich (219g)	563	293	28	39	33	88	1108	
Cheeseburger, large, single patty, with ham, condiments and vegetables 1 sandwich (254g)	744	430	41	38	48	122	1712	

Food Serving size	Cal.	Fat cal.	Prot.	Carb.	Fat	Chol.	Sod.	Fiber
Cheeseburger, regular, double patty and bun, plain 1 sandwich (160g)	461	200	22	45	22	80	891	
Cheeseburger, regular, double patty and bun, with condiments and vegetables 1 sandwich (228g)	650	305	30	52	34	93	921	
Cheeseburger, regular, double patty, plain 1 sandwich (155g)	457	249	28	22	28	110	636	
Cheeseburger, regular, double patty, with condiments and vegetables 1 sandwich (166g)	417	192	22	35	22	60	1051	
Cheeseburger, regular, single meat patty, plain 1 sandwich (102g)	319	135	14	32	15	50	500	
Cheeseburger, regular, single patty, with condiments and vegetables 1 sandwich (154g)	359	176	18	28	20	52	976	
Cheeseburger, regular, single patty, with condiments 1 sandwich (113g)	295	129	16	26	15	37	616	
Cheeseburger, triple patty, plain 1 sandwich (304g)	796	461	55	27	52	161	1213	
Chicken fillet sandwich, plain 1 sandwich (182g)	515	259	24	38	29	60	957	
Chicken fillet sandwich, with cheese 1 sandwich (228g)	632	345	30	41	39	78	1238	
Chicken, breaded and fried, boneless pieces, plain 1 piece (18g)	49		3	3	3	10	87	0.0
Chicken, breaded and fried, boneless pieces, with barbecue sauce 6 pieces (130g)	330	161	17	25	18	61	829	
Chicken, breaded and fried, boneless pieces, with honey 6 pieces (115g)	329	153	17	26	17	61	537	
Chicken, breaded and fried, boneless pieces, with mustard sauce 6 pieces (130g)	322	172	17	21	20	61	790	
Chicken, breaded and fried, boneless pieces, with sweet and sour sauce 6 pieces (130g)	346	162	17	29	18	61	677	
Chicken, breaded and fried, dark meat (drumstick or thigh) 2 pieces (148g)	431	240	30	16	27	166	755	

Food Serving size	Cal.	Fat cal.	Prot.	Carb.	Fat	Chol.	Sod.	Fiber
Chicken, breaded and fried, light meat (breast or wing)								
2 pieces (163g)	494	265	36	20	29	148	975	
Chili con carne								
1 cup (8 fl oz) (253g)	256	68	25	23	8	134	1007	
Chili with Beans								
1 cup (253g)	412	228	18	28	25	56	1171	10.1
Chili without Beans								
1 cup (250g)	430	293	18	18	33	85	1588	2.5
Chimichanga, with beef and cheese								
1 chimichanga (183g)	443	209	20	38	24	51	957	
Chimichanga, with beef and red chili peppers								
1 chimichanga (190g)	424	171	19	46	19	10	1169	
Chimichanga, with beef, cheese, and red chili peppers								
1 chimichanga (180g)	364	158	14	38	18	50	895	
Chimichanga, with beef								
1 chimichanga (174g)	425	168	19	44	19	9	910	
Clams, breaded and fried								
¾ cup (115g)	451	237	13	39	26	87	834	
Coleslaw								
¾ cup (99g)	147	95	1	13	11	5	267	
Cookies, animal crackers								
1 box (67g)	299	73	4	50	9	11	273	
Cookies, chocolate chip								
1 box (55g)	233	98	3	36	12	12	188	
Corn on the cob with butter								
1 ear (146g)	155	25	4	32	3	6	29	
Corned Beef Hash								
1 cup (253g)	486	273	25	28	30	89	1594	5.1
Crab cake								
1 cake (60g)	160	91	11	5	10	82	491	0.0
Crab, baked								
1 crab (109g)	160	19	28	4	2	184	549	0.0
Crab, soft-shell, fried								
1 crab (125g)	334	157	11	31	18	45	1118	

Food Serving size	Cal.	Fat cal.	Prot.	Carb.	Fat	Chol.	Sod.	Fiber
Croissant, with egg and cheese 1 croissant (127g)	368	213	13	24	24	216	551	
Croissant, with egg, cheese, and bacon 1 croissant (129g)	413	251	17	23	28	215	889	
Croissant, with egg, cheese, and ham 1 croissant (152g)	474	297	18	24	33	213	1081	
Croissant, with egg, cheese, and sausage 1 croissant (160g)	523	341	21	24	38	216	1115	
Danish pastry, cheese 1 pastry (91g)	353	216	5	29	25	20	319	
Danish pastry, cinnamon 1 pastry (88g)	349	147	4	47	17	27	326	
Danish pastry, fruit 1 pastry (94g)	335	141	5	45	16	19	333	
Deli Franks 1 serving (45g)	112	57	10	4	6	0	431	2.7
Egg and cheese sandwich 1 sandwich (146g)	340	168	16	26	19	291	804	
Egg, scrambled 2 eggs (94g)	199	134	13	2	15	400	211	0.0
Enchilada, with cheese and beef 1 enchilada (192g)	323	152	12	31	17	40	1319	
Enchilada, with cheese 1 enchilada (163g)	319	172	10	29	20	44	784	
Enchirito, with cheese, beef, and beans 1 enchilada or enchirito (193g)	344	136	17	35	15	50	1251	
English muffin, with butter 1 muffin (63g)	189	50	5	30	6	13	386	
English muffin, with cheese and sausage 1 muffin (115g)	393	215	15	29	24	59	1036	1.1
English muffin, with egg, cheese, and Canadian bacon 1 sandwich (137g)	289		16	27	12	234	729	1.4
English muffin, with egg, cheese, and sausage 1 muffin (165g)	487	279	21	31	31	274	1135	

Food Serving size	Cal.	Fat cal.	Prot.	Carb.	Fat	Chol.	Sod.	Fiber
Fish fillet, battered or breaded, and fried 1 fillet (91g)	211	96	14	15	11	31	484	0.0
Fish sandwich, with tartar sauce and cheese 1 sandwich (183g)	523	258	20	48	29	68	939	
Fish sandwich, with tartar sauce 1 sandwich (158g)	431	194	17	41	22	55	615	
Flame broiled cutlet shaped chicken patty with honey mustard sauce 1 piece (85g)	167		18	8	7	47	611	0.9
Flame broiled cutlet shaped chicken patty with teriyaki sauce 1 piece (85g)	165		18	8	7	47	576	0.9
French toast sticks 5 pieces (141g)	513	261	8	58	30	75	499	2.8
French toast with butter 2 slices (135g)	356	167	11	36	19	116	513	
Fried pie, fruit (apple, cherry, or lemon) 1 fried pie (5″ × 3¾″) (85g)	266	129	3	33	14	13	325	
Frijoles with cheese 1 cup (167g)	225	73	12	28	8	37	882	
Frozen bagel french toast with maple syrup 1 serving (71g)	190		14	21	6	129	283	0.0
Ham and cheese sandwich 1 sandwich (146g)	352	141	20	34	16	58	771	
Ham, egg, and cheese sandwich 1 sandwich (143g)	347	140	19	31	16	246	1005	
Hamburger, large, double patty, with condiments and vegetables 1 sandwich (226g)	540	242	34	41	27	122	791	
Hamburger, large, single meat patty, plain 1 sandwich (137g)	426	208	23	32	23	71	474	
Hamburger, large, single meat patty, with condiments and vegetables 1 sandwich (218g)	512	254	26	39	28	87	824	
Hamburger, large, single patty, with condiments 1 sandwich (172g)	427		22	36	21	71	731	1.7

Food Serving size	Cal.	Fat cal.	Prot.	Carb.	Fat	Chol.	Sod.	Fiber
Hamburger, large, triple patty, with condiments 1 sandwich (259g)	692	370	49	28	41	142	712	
Hamburger, double patty, plain 1 sandwich (176g)	544	251	30	42	28	99	554	
Hamburger, double patty, with condiments 1 sandwich (215g)	576	288	32	39	32	103	742	
Hamburger, single patty, plain 1 sandwich (90g)	275	103	13	31	12	35	387	
Hamburger, single patty, with condiments and vegetables 1 sandwich (110g)	279	116	13	28	13	26	504	
Hamburger, single patty, with condiments 1 sandwich (106g)	272		13	34	10	30	534	2.1
Hot dog, plain 1 sandwich (98g)	242	131	11	18	15	44	670	
Hot dog, with chili 1 sandwich (114g)	296	122	14	31	14	51	480	
Hot dog, with corn flour coating (corndog) 1 sandwich (175g)	460	172	18	56	19	79	973	
Hush puppies 5 pieces (78g)	257	103	5	35	12	135	965	
Ice milk, vanilla, soft-serve, with cone 1 cone (103g)	164	54	4	24	6	28	92	0.0
Macaroni and cheese 1 cup (253g)	283	91	10	35	10	28	1343	2.5
Nachos, with cheese and jalapeno peppers 6–8 nachos (204g)	608	297	16	59	35	84	1736	
Nachos, with cheese, beans, ground beef, and peppers 6–8 nachos (255g)	569	261	20	56	31	20	1800	
Nachos, with cheese 6–8 nachos (113g)	346	163	9	36	19	18	816	
Nachos, with cinnamon and sugar 6–8 nachos (109g)	592	305	8	63	36	39	439	
Onion rings, breaded and fried 8–9 onion rings (83g)	276	139	3	32	16	14	430	

Food Serving size	Cal.	Fat cal.	Prot.	Carb.	Fat	Chol.	Sod.	Fiber
Oysters, battered or breaded, and fried 6 pieces (139g)	368	162	13	40	18	108	677	
Pancakes with butter and syrup 2 cakes (232g)	520	122	9	90	14	58	1104	
Pizza with cheese, meat, and vegetables 1 slice (79g)	184	49	13	21	6	21	382	
Pizza with cheese 1 slice (63g)	140	28	8	21	3	9	336	
Pizza with pepperoni 1 slice (71g)	181	63	10	20	7	14	267	
Potato salad $\frac{1}{3}$ cup (95g)	108	51	2	13	6	57	312	
Potato, baked and topped with cheese sauce and bacon 1 piece (299g)	451	235	18	45	27	30	972	
Potato, baked and topped with cheese sauce and broccoli 1 piece (339g)	403	179	14	47	20	20	485	
Potato, baked and topped with cheese sauce and chili 1 piece (395g)	482	209	24	55	24	32	699	
Potato, baked and topped with cheese sauce 1 piece (296g)	474	261	15	47	30	18	382	
Potato, baked and topped with sour cream and chives 1 piece (302g)	393	186	6	51	21	24	181	
Potato, French fried in vegetable oil 1 medium (134g)	409		5	52	20	0	265	5.4
Potato, mashed $\frac{1}{3}$ cup (80g)	66	7	2	13	1	2	182	
Potatoes, hashed brown $\frac{1}{2}$ cup (72g)	151	82	2	16	9	9	290	
Pre-cooked frozen egg and cheese biscuit sandwich 1 serving (99g)	224		10	25	9	111	563	0.0
Pre-cooked frozen egg and cheese pockets 1 serving (64g)	147		7	15	8	93	233	1.3
Pre-cooked frozen egg, ham and cheese biscuit sandwich 1 serving (120g)	242		12	25	10	114	722	0.0

Food Serving size	Cal.	Fat cal.	Prot.	Carb.	Fat	Chol.	Sod.	Fiber
Roast beef sandwich with cheese 1 sandwich (176g)	473	155	32	46	18	77	1633	
Roast beef sandwich, plain 1 sandwich (139g)	346	124	21	33	14	51	792	
Salad, vegetable, tossed, without dressing, with cheese and egg 1.5 cups (217g)	102	57	9	4	7	98	119	
Salad, vegetable, tossed, without dressing, with chicken 1.5 cups (218g)	105	20	17	4	2	72	209	
Salad, vegetable, tossed, without dressing, with pasta and seafood 1.5 cups (417g)	379	183	17	33	21	50	1572	
Salad, vegetable, tossed, without dressing, with shrimp 1.5 cups (236g)	106	21	14	7	2	179	489	
Salad, vegetable, tossed, without dressing $\frac{3}{4}$ cup (104g)	17	0	1	3	0	0	27	
Salad, vegetables tossed, without dressing, with turkey, ham and cheese 1.5 cups (326g)	267	144	26	3	16	140	743	
Scallops, breaded and fried 6 pieces (144g)	386	165	16	39	19	108	919	
Shrimp, breaded and fried 6–8 shrimp (164g)	454	219	20	39	25	200	1446	
Spaghetti Bolognese, frozen entree 1 serving (283g)	255	25	14	42	3	17	473	5.7
Spicy black bean burger 1 patty (78g)	115		12	15	1	1	499	4.7
Spicy chili with beans 1 cup (253g)	423	228	18	33	25	56	1485	5.1
Steak sandwich 1 sandwich (204g)	459	128	31	51	14	73	798	
Submarine sandwich, with cold cuts 1 submarine (228g)	456	161	23	50	18	36	1651	
Submarine sandwich, with roast beef 1 submarine (216g)	410	116	28	45	13	73	845	

Food Serving size	Cal.	Fat cal.	Prot.	Carb.	Fat	Chol.	Sod.	Fiber
Submarine sandwich, with tuna salad								
1 submarine (256g)	584	246	31	56	28	49	1293	
Sundae, caramel								
1 sundae (155g)	304	82	8	50	9	25	195	0.0
Sundae, hot fudge								
1 sundae (158g)	284	69	6	47	8	21	182	0.0
Sundae, strawberry								
1 sundae (153g)	268	67	6	44	8	21	92	0.0
Taco salad with chili con carne								
1.5 cups (261g)	290	114	18	26	13	5	885	
Taco salad								
1.5 cups (198g)	279	121	14	24	14	44	762	
Taco								
1 small (171g)	369	180	21	27	21	56	802	
Tostada with guacamole								
2 pieces (261g)	360	198	13	31	23	39	799	
Tostada, with beans and cheese								
1 piece (144g)	223	86	10	26	10	30	543	
Tostada, with beans, beef, and cheese								
1 piece (225g)	333	157	16	29	18	74	871	
Tostada, with beef and cheese								
1 piece (163g)	315	143	20	23	16	41	897	
Vegetable patties								
1 patty (67g)	119	36	11	10	4	1	382	4.0
Wrapped breakfast sandwich with cheese								
1 piece (92g)	236		11	26	11	26	677	1.8
Wrapped ham breakfast sandwich								
1 piece (95g)	223		11	26	9	26	660	1.9
Wrapped sausage breakfast sandwich								
1 piece (89g)	263		12	26	13	22	495	1.8